Superficial Keratitis

Monographs in Ophthalmology 1

Dr. W. JUNK bv PUBLISHERS THE HAGUE – BOSTON – LONDON

Superficial Keratitis

Edited by

P.C. MAUDGAL and L. MISSOTTEN

The Eye Research Laboratory and
the Ophthalmological Clinic
Catholic University of Leuven, Belgium

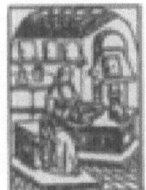

Dr. W. JUNK bv PUBLISHERS THE HAGUE – BOSTON – LONDON

REPRINTED FROM Bull. Soc. belge Ophtal. 187-I, 1980

Distributors:

for the United States and Canada

Kluwer Boston Inc.
190 Old Derby Street
Hingham, MA 02043
USA

for all other countries

Kluwer Academic Publishing Group
Distribution Center
P.O. Box 322
3300 AH Dordrecht
The Netherlands

ISBN-13: 978-94-009-8673-2   e-ISBN-13: 978-94-009-8671 -8
DOI:10.1007/978-94-009-8671-8

CONTENTS

PREFACE

In its long series of annual reports, the Belgian Society of Ophthalmology has a tradition of bringing into focus the recent advances in ophthalmology. But it seems surprising that one has to go back to 1940 to find a major report on the corneal diseases, when R. Rubbrecht wrote an "Aperçu de la pathologie et de la therapeutique générale des maladies de la cornée". However, this omission is only apparent. In fact, many reports, since then, have contributed to our knowledge of the advances in corneal research.

The corneal dimensions were documented in "La biometrie oculaire clinique (Y. Delmarcelle et al., 1976)", the fine structure of the cornea in "L'ultrastructure de tissues oculaires (L. Missotten, 1964)", and many aspects of its metabolism in "Les verres de contact (P. Cochet et al, 1967)" and "Les complications oculaires des erreurs congenitales du metabolism (J.P. Groux et O. Kallay, 1971)".

Bacterial keratitis was a main topic in "La therapeutique par les antibiotiques autres que la Penicillamine en Ophtalmologie (J. Michiels, 1952). Fungal corneal infections were described in detail in "Les mycoses oculaires" (J . François et M. Elewaut-Rysselaere, 1968)" and the toxic effects of drugs were dealt with in "Les effets nocifs des médications générales sur l'appareil visuel (J. Michiels et coll. 1972)".

This report is mainly concerned with the diseases of the superficial corneal layer which forms the most important surface in the optical system of the eye. Our aim has not been to present an encyclopedic review of the superficial corneal diseases of diverse etiology, but to discuss at length the common disorders of the epithelium, and other relevant conditions important in the differential diagnosis of superficial keratitis. Congenital anomalies, corneal involvement in systemic disorders, dystrophies of the cornea, and the fungal and bacterial keratitis are not dealt with in this report.

Our many colleagues and friends, referred their patients with unusual superficial corneal lesions to us. To name them individually will be an endless task. We are deeply endebted to them. Mrs. C. Van

Rymenant did the tedious job of typing the manuscript and provided secretarial help, and Mrs. A. Geysen's technical assistance was invaluable in the laboratory. They deserve our sincere thanks.

We are also grateful to the Catholic University of Leuven (KUL) and the National Fund for Medical Scientific Research (NFGWO) for their support of the investigations on corneal diseases.

Last, but not the least, we thank the Executive Board of the Belgisch Oftalmologisch Gezelschap, Nederlandstalige afdeling (Belgian Society of Ophthalmology, Dutch language division), for entrusting this report to us.

CHAPTER I

DIAGNOSTIC TECHNIQUES IN SUPERFICIAL KERATITIS

"Greater is thine own task, even if this be humble, than the task of another, even if this be great. When a man does the duty imposed upon him by his own nature, no sin can touch this man".

Bhagavad Gita XVIII. 47

The nature of our profession makes it our prime duty to preserve vision and combat eye disease by making diagnosis and instituting appropriate therapy. To achieve this goal, one begins with history taking followed by clinical examination of the patient to detect signs of a specific illness. On the basis of this investigation, during which some specific clinical tests may have to be performed, one arrives at the diagnosis of disease, i.e. the physician has recognized the cause of illness. Additional laboratory tests may help to confirm the clinical diagnosis.

The art of history taking and the principles and methods of clinical examination are described in standard text and reference books on the diseases of the eye. We shall describe here only the laboratory investigations applicable in the diagnosis of superficial keratitis.

Scrapings and smears

Scrapings may be obtained by a cleaned sterile platinum spatula or loop, the blade of a knife or a cotton-tip-applicator. No anesthetic is required in obtaining material from the lid margins and conjunctiva, while topical anesthetic should be instilled before scraping the cornea. Conjunctival scrapings are generally taken from lower palpebral conjunctiva and fornix; but if a localized disease under upper eyelid is suspected, it is imperative to obtain material from the involved site.

The material obtained from swabbings or scrapings is smeared on clean glass slides which may be either air dried or fixed with a suitable fixative depending upon the staining one wishes to perform. In routine laboratory work Gram or Giemsa stainings are very useful. Methanol fixation of the material is required for both of these techniques. Gram stain is mainly used to detect the presence of various Gram positive and negative bacteria while Giemsa stain is more suitable for cytological work and detection of fungi. The study of the inflammatory cellular response gives clues to the viral or allergic nature of the disease, if no micro-organisms are detected. Polymorphonuclear leukocytes are abundant in bacterial, fungal and chlamydial infections, while lymphocytes are predominant in viral infections. An increased number of eosinophils indicates an allergic disorder. Cytoplasmic and nuclear inclusions develop in a number of viral infections.

Different staining procedures (including immunofluorescent methods) have been developed to detect the presence of specific micro organisms in the smears.

Cultures

Material for cultures is obtained in a similar way as for smears. Material from conjunctiva is generally obtained with a cotton-tip-applicator moistened with nutrient broth and a spatula may be necessary to scrape material from a corneal lesion or lid margin. Dry swabs used to obtain culture material give a lesser yield of bacteria than the wet swabs. It is better to inoculate the material directly into culture plates and in the broth. Cultures should be done to detect the aerobic and anaerobic bacteria at the same time. If fungus infection is suspected Sabourauds' medium should be used. Special cell-culture systems are needed to grow viruses.

Corneal replicas

Scrapings of the cornea have one major disadvantage that they destroy the histological pattern of the corneal lesions. We developed the corneal replica technique (Missotten and Maudgal, 1977; Maudgal, 1978) to overcome this difficulty. The results obtained till now with this technique are described under specific disease conditions. This method did not produce any damage or complications in more than 150 human eyes where it was used. Moreover, making a corneal replica heals many forms of superficial keratitis.

Technique

A topical anesthetic is instilled into the eye. The eyelids are kept open with a speculum. The cornea is dried by blowing air for about one minute (fig. I-1a). An airpump used in fish-tanks is suitable for this purpose and easy to handle. After drying the precorneal tearfilm a viscous solution of collodion in amyl acetate is painted on the corneal surface from where a replica is desired (fig. I-1b). Originally we used concentrations of 2.15 to 2.3% collodion in amyl acetate. Subsequent experience has shown that dry collodion supplied by different firms does not give consistent viscosity in equal concentrations and the solution may not be transparent. The amount of collodion in solutions prepared from different batches varies. One may have to reach concentration of 4% or higher to obtain the desired viscosity. A solution of good viscosity should be easy to paint but should not drop from the brush or flow away from the area of application. Turbid solutions are unsuitable for microscopic study of the replicas.

The solution painted on the cornea is dried by blowing air for about 2 minutes (fig. I-1c). As the solution dries it develops fine furrows like ripples. The collodion membrane so formed on the cornea is caught at the margin with a fine curved forceps and peeled off (fig. I-1d). Generally the whole membrane is removed in toto. If it breaks and some part is left on the cornea, it falls off spontaneously in one or two days without any harm to the eye.

The lid speculum is removed and the eye is patched. The patch is left undisturbed for two days without applying any medication. The epithelial wound made by the replica heals in 2 to 4 days.

The collodion membrane is mounted on glass slides in 0,1% albumin or gelatin, keeping epithelium side down. A piece of paper inserted between the plastic cover slip and the replica prevents sticking of the replica to the cover slip. The slides may be dried in an oven or at room temperature. The coverslip and the underlying paper are removed while the replica remains sticking on the slide. It can be studied by phase contrast and oblique illumination microscopy. One needs some experience in the interpretation of the microscopic picture as small air-bubbles and dust may produce many artefacts. However, the microscopic picture becomes clear if the flat mounts of

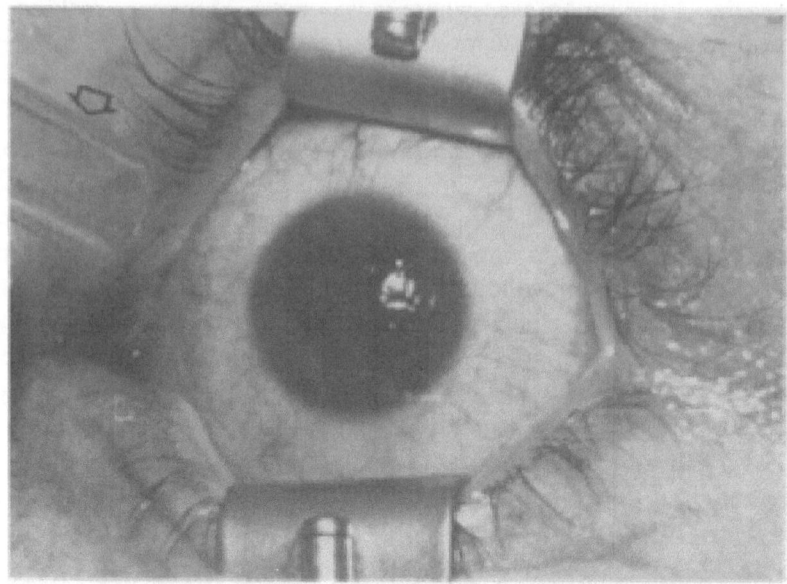

Fig. I-1a. — Air is blown on the cornea through a tubing (arrow) connected to an air-pump.

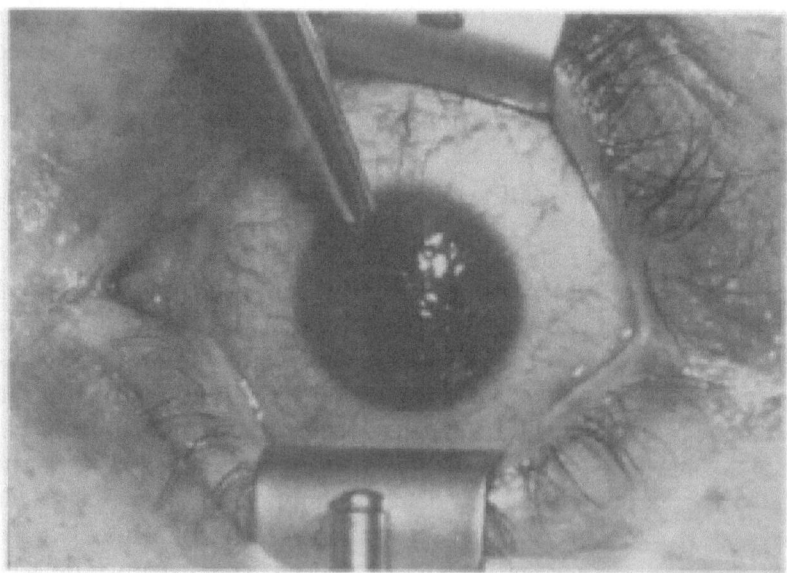

Fig. I-1b. — Collodion in amyl acetate solution is painted on the dried cornea.

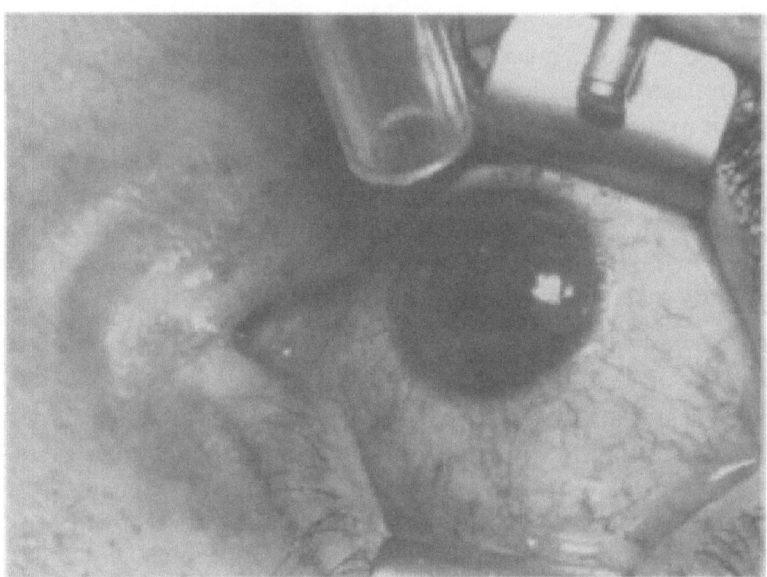

Fig. I-1c. — Air is blown again to dry the painted solution.

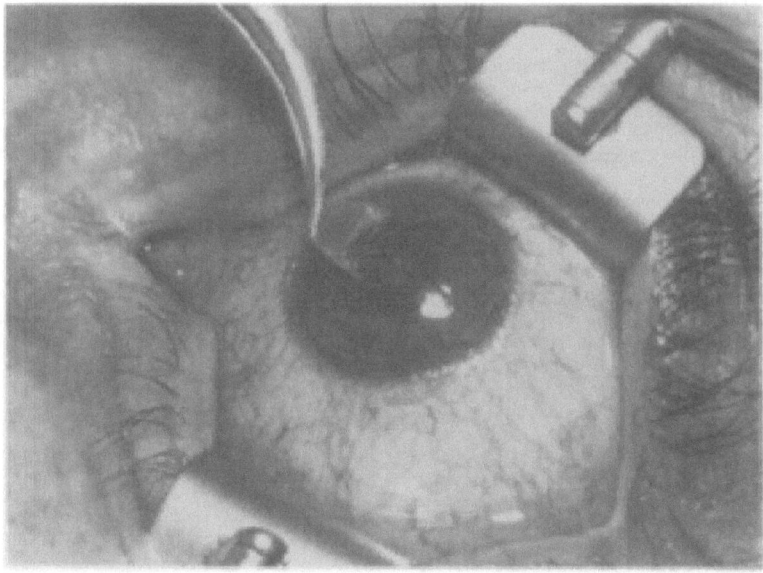

Fig. I-1d. — The collodion membrane is peeled off.

cells are studied after dissolving the collodion membrane in acetone. Cytological, histochemical and immunofluorescent stainings can be done on such preparations.

For electron microscopy the replicas are fixed in buffered glutaraldehyde and processed further like biopsy specimens. Difficulties, however, arise to locate the cells in the embedded epoxy resin for sectioning. This is especially true if only a few cells have been removed with the replica. Currently, we are trying to modify the embedding techniques to overcome this problem.

Serological tests

Serological tests are available for detection of different bacterial and viral infections. Acute and convalescent sera should be tested to detect a four-fold increase in the antibody titers. A single positive examination indicates exposure to the specific micro organisms in the past while the absence of antibodies in serum rules out the possibility of exposure.

FURTHER READING

Aronson, S.B. and Elliot, J.H. — Ocular inflammation. The C.V. Mosby Company, St. Louis, 1972.
Fedukowicz, H.B. — External infections of the eye. Appleton-Century-Crofts, New York, 1978.
Keeney, A.H. — Ocular examination, basis and technique. The C.V. Mosby Company, St. Louis, 1976.
Locatcher-Khorazo, D. and Seegal, B.C. — Microbiology of the eye. The C.V. Mosby Company, 1972.
Norn, M.S. — External Eye, methods of examination. Scripter, Copenhagen, 1974.

BIBLIOGRAPHY

Missotten, L. and Maudgal, P.C. — The replica technique used to study superficial corneal epithelium in vivo. *Amer. J. Ophthal.*, *84*, 104, 1977.
Maudgal, P.C. — The epithelial response in keratitis sicca and keratitis herpetica. *Doctoral thesis*, University of Leuven, 1976. *Doc. Ophthalmologica*, *45*, 223, 1978.

CHAPTER II

THE CORNEA

The cornea is the anterior transparent part of the outer coat of the eye. At its periphery it continues into the opaque sclera. The transitional zone between the cornea and sclera is termed limbus.

Viewed from outside the cornea is elliptical in shape, its major horizontal axis being 11-12 mm long in most of the eyes. When viewed from inside the cornea is perfectly circular. The corneal diameter is 1% larger in males than in females. Measured by in vivo pachometry in humans the central cornea is 0.56 ± 0.04 mm thick (Delmarcelle et. al., 1976). Its thickness depends upon the osmolarity of tears, temperature, oxygen supply, drug therapy and age. In the limbal region the cornea is somewhat thicker i.e. 0.67 mm at middle age.

Due to its transparency and refractive index the cornea serves as the major lens of the optical system of the eye. Its refractive power depends on its curvature and the index of refraction. The radius of curvature of its outer surface is 7.86 ± 0.26 mm (Prijot et al., 1964) and its refractive index is 1.376. This produces a refractive power of 38.8 D in the anterior central region of the cornea. A variation of curvature from 7.0 to 8.5 mm is compatible with good visual function. Again, in males the radius is $\pm 1.5\%$ larger than in females.

Histology

We shall briefly consider the histology and ultrastructure of the cornea in relation to the physiological function. The cornea can be roughly subdivided into the anterior and posterior limiting layers enclosing the stroma or substantia propria.

The anterior limiting layers are further subdivided into the epithelium, basement membrane and in primates the Bowman's membrane. The posterior limiting layers are formed by the Descemet's membrane and endothelium. On its outer surface the cornea is bathed by tear film. Since the tear film plays an important role in the normal physiology and function of the cornea, it is not inappropriate to include a short description of this fluid layer here.

Tear film

The tear film constantly bathes the outer surface of the cornea. The unstained tearfilm is invisible on the cornea but with the slit lamp a strip of tears is normally seen between the eyeball and lid margin. The film is constantly renewed by the secretions of tear producing glands. The tear film serves an optical function by filling the tiny irregularities in the corneal surface. At the same time it lubricates the outer eye making the smooth mechanical lid movements possible. Small foreign bodies and the cell debris are either flushed away by the aqueous film or they are trapped in the conjunctival mucus and removed. Tears have some antibacterial properties by virtue of their lysozyme content. Diffusion of oxygen from the atmosphere to the cornea takes place through this layer.

Three distinct component layers are recognised in the tear film.

The superficial layer is composed of oily secretions of the meibomian glands and the accessory sebacious glands of Zeiss. Both types of these glands are located in the lids. The oily layer reduces the

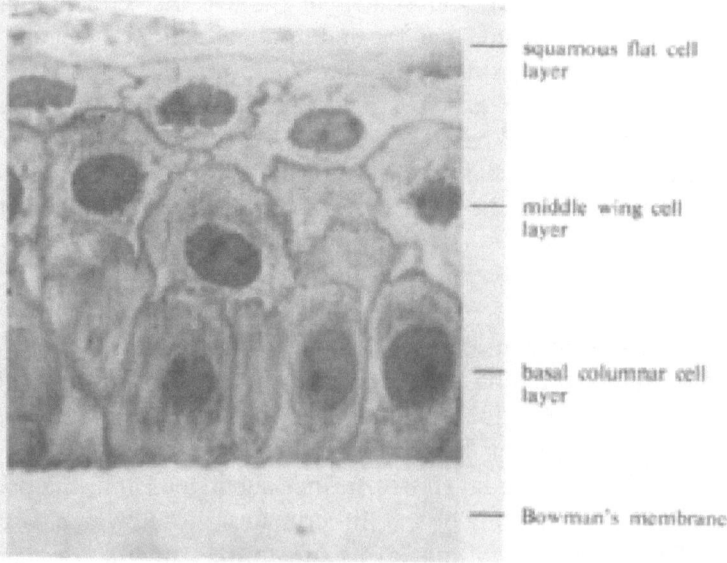

squamous flat cell layer

middle wing cell layer

basal columnar cell layer

Bowman's membrane

Fig. II-1. — Histological section of the human corneal epithelium Toluidine blue stain × 915.

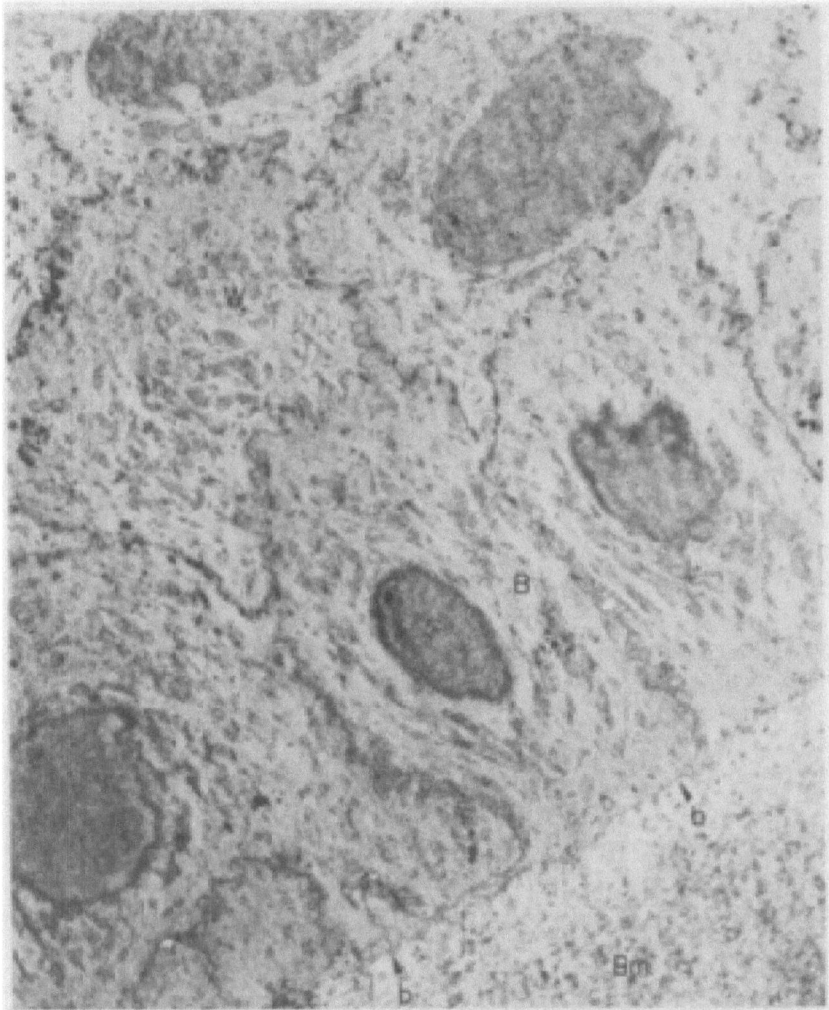

Fig. II-2. — Transmission electron microscopy of human cornea shows interdigitations of cell membranes. Intercellular spaces are absent. The attachments of the basal columnar cells (B) to the basement membrane (b) are flat. W = wing cells, Bm = Bowman's membrane. × 4150.

evaporation of subjacent aqueous layer. It also prevents the overflow of tears along the lid margins by increasing the surface tension. Reduction of oily secretions as in chronic meibomianitis may lead to decreased tear film break-up time and dry spots on the cornea.

The middle aqueous layer is 6.5 to 7.5 µ thick. It is formed by the secretions of the lacrimal gland and the accessory glands of Krause

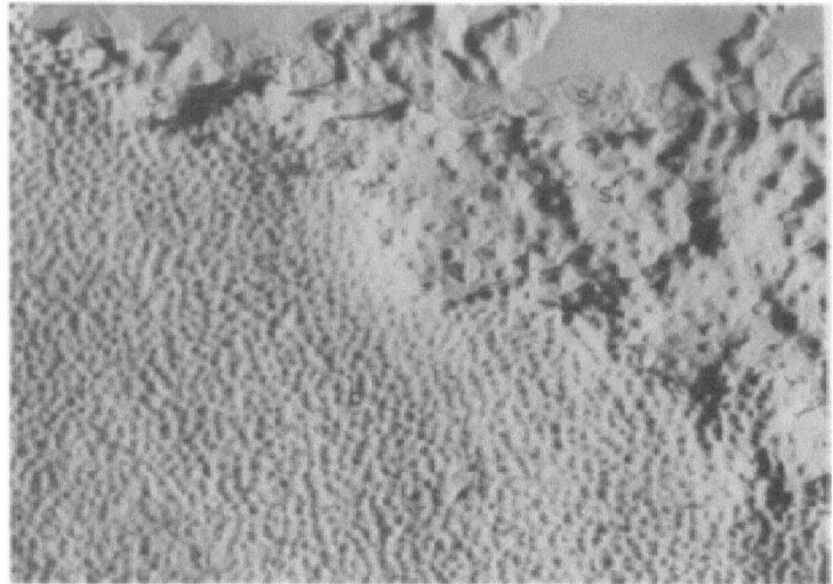

Fig. II-3. — Flat preparation of rabbit corneal epithelium mounted upside down. b = basal cells; S′ = the row of squamous cells under superficial cells; S = superficial cells. Oblique illumination microscopy. × 225.

and Wolfring. The latter glands are located in the eye lids while the lacrimal gland occupies the shallow lacrimal fossa under the upper temporal orbital rim, between the globe and the lateral process of the frontal bone.

Deficiency of the aqueous component of tear film generally results in dry eyes.

The deepest layer of the tear film is formed by the mucus secretion of conjunctival goblet cells and crypts of Henle in the fornices. By adsorption on the hydrophobic corneal epithelium the mucus layer renders it hydrophillic so that it becomes wettable. Decreased mucoid secretion can lead to dry eye conditions even in the presence of adequate aqueous tear secretion.

In clinical practice the quantity of tear secretion can be measured by Schirmer's test and other more sophisticated tests. In the presence of adequate tear secretion, decreased tear film break-up time may indicate a reduction of the oily or mucus layers. These tests are described in detail in the chapter on dry eyes.

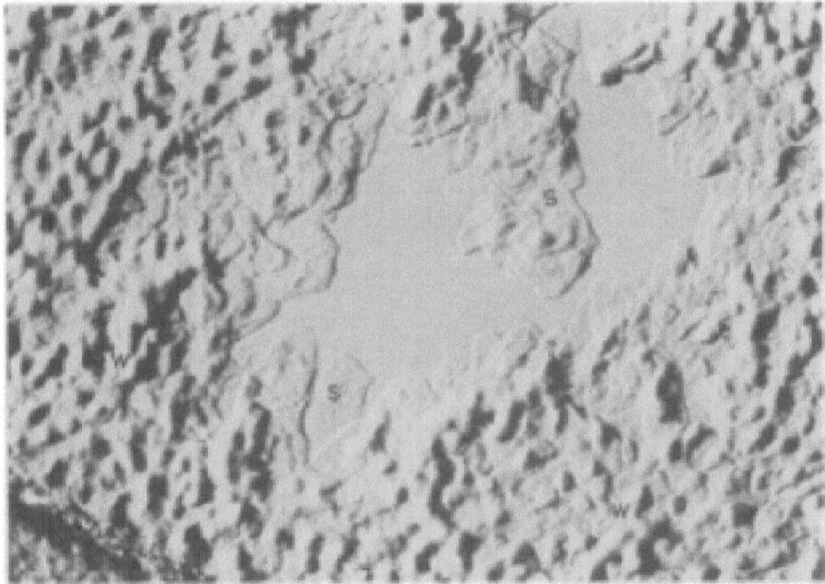

Fig. II-4. — Flat mount of rabbit corneal epithelium mounted upside down shows undersurface of wing cells (W) and superficial cells (S). Oblique illumination microscopy. × 300.

Epithelium

The epithelium of the human cornea is about $50\,\mu$ thick. It is made of 5 to 6 layers of cells (fig. II-1). The cells of the deepest layer, the basal layer, are columnar in shape. Their attachments to the basement membrane are flat (fig. II-2). However, if flat preparations of the epithelium are viewed upside down, the rabbit basal cell nuclei appear forming rounded protrusions (fig. II-3). The upper end of each cell is also rounded. Slightly elongated nuclei are situated more towards the apical part of the cells. Some cells in this layer stain more intensely with different stains and appear more electron dense in the electron microscope. Teng (1961) ascribed a secretory function to such cells. In some disease conditions like keratoconus (Teng, 1961) and dry eyes (Maudgal, 1978) these cells increase in number. Like all other cells, Teng cells migrate outwards and flatten out to become polyhedral wing cells of the middle layer. This layer is 2 to 3 cells thick (figs. II-1; II-2 and II-4). The cells contain rounded nuclei in the center. Further outward migration is accompanied by increased flattening until they become squamous cells of the superficial layer (figs. II-1; II-3; II-4 and II-5). Their nuclei and cytoplasmic organelles become indistinct but flat mounts of superficial cells have shown that these cells still possess nuclei which protrude on the surface in dehydrated specimens (Missotten and Maudgal, 1977; Maudgal and Missotten, 1978). Some cells are binucleate and rarely trinucleate. The nuclei may have crenated margins with clumping of nuclear chromatin. Sex chromatin may be detected in some cells (fig. II-6).

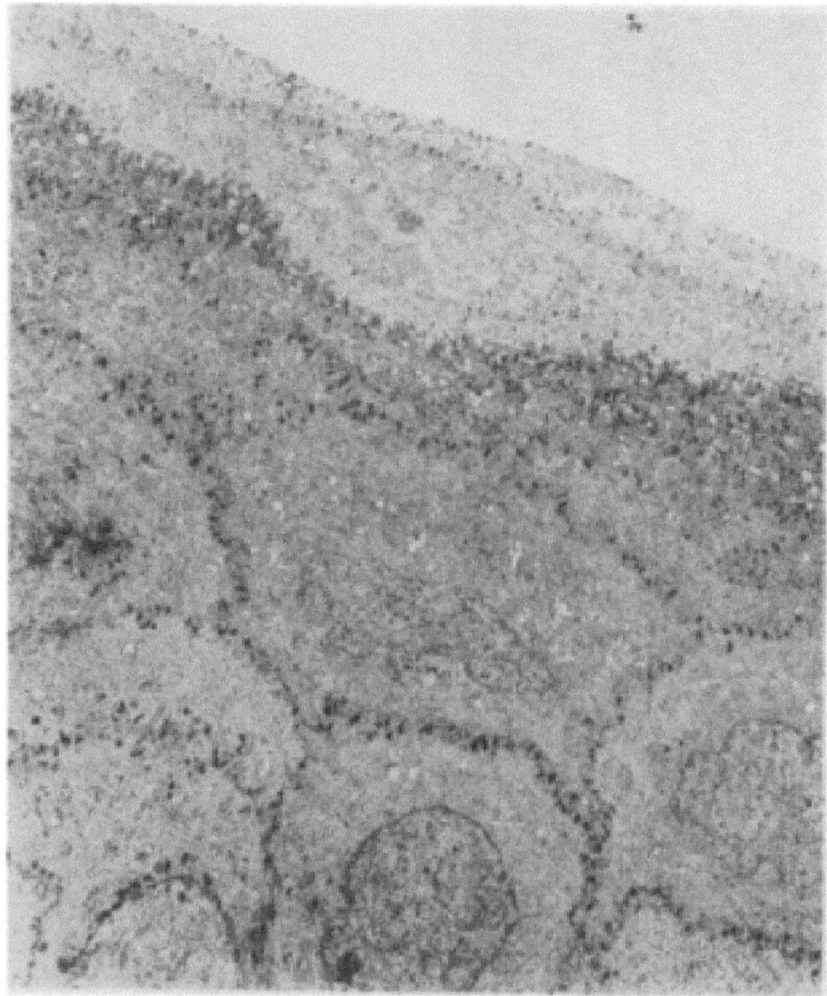

Fig. II-5. — Transmission electron microscopy of human corneal epithelium showing middle wing cell layer and upper squamous cell layer. × 4150.

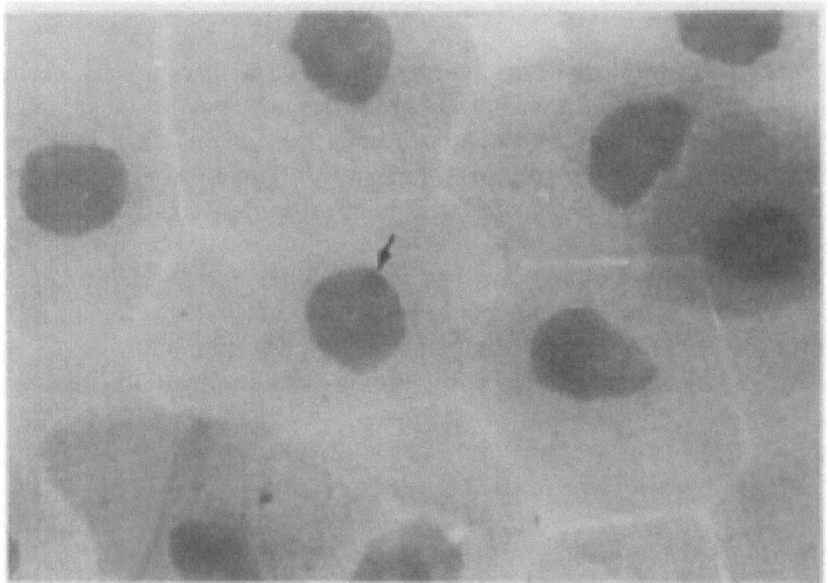

Fig. II-6. — Sex chromatin in a nucleus (arrow). Flat mount of rabbit superficial epithelium by replica technique. Toluidine blue ammonium molybdate stain. ×900.

Cytoplasmic vacuoles are often observed. The cell borders are generally neatly apposed but there may be slight overlapping of smaller borders. These cells are in a state of gradual metabolic shut-down and eventually shed off from the corneal surface. Shedding seems to take place in patches.

Structural proteins of the epithelium

Corneal epithelial cells are relatively tough cells due to their structural protein contents. Reticulin is present in the epithelial cells (Maudgal, 1978; Maudgal and Missotten, 1978). Although superficial cells do not keratinize under normal conditions, the intracellular electron dense tonofibril bundles gradually increase during the migration of the cells from basal to the superficial layers. Actual keratinization of the cells takes place under dry eye conditions, probably as a protective response to conserve water (Maudgal, 1978).

Recently, actin filaments have been demonstrated in the corneal epithelium cells (Gipson and Anderson, 1977, Rahi and Ashton, 1978). This contractile protein may help in the migration of cells in the healing of corneal erosions.

Cell membranes

The cell membranes form interdigitations with adjacent cells which are attached to each other by numerous desmosomes, or attachment bodies (figs. II-2 and II-7). The columnar cells of the basal layer are attached to the basement membrane by asymmetrical or hemidesmosomes with the basement membrane forming half of the structure.

Intercellular spaces are few, the cell membranes are in close apposition. The epithelium offers, therefore, an effective barrier against diffusion of fluid. In the rabbit, removal of the epithelium produces an excess hydration of the corneal stroma, resulting in 200% increase in the corneal thickness in 24 hours. Dissolved substances penetrate slowly through the epithelium, unless they have a high lipid and aqueous solubility.

Metabolic equipment

The rapid turn over of the cells and the well known rapid healing of defects in the epithelium suggest that these cells have a high

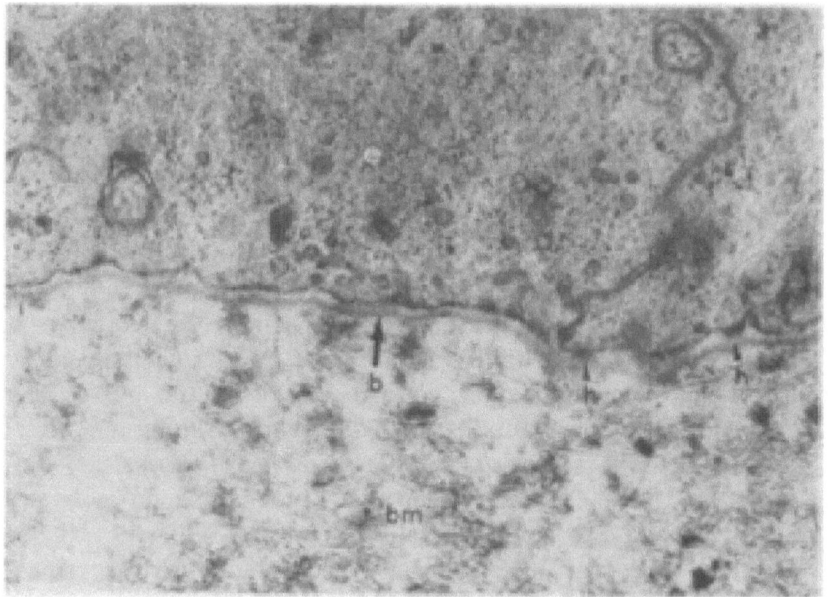

Fig. II-7. — Transmission electron microscopy of human corneal epithelium. *e* = basal epithelium cells; *h* = hemidesmosomal attachments; *b* = basement membrane; *bm* = Bowman's membrane. × 21 375.

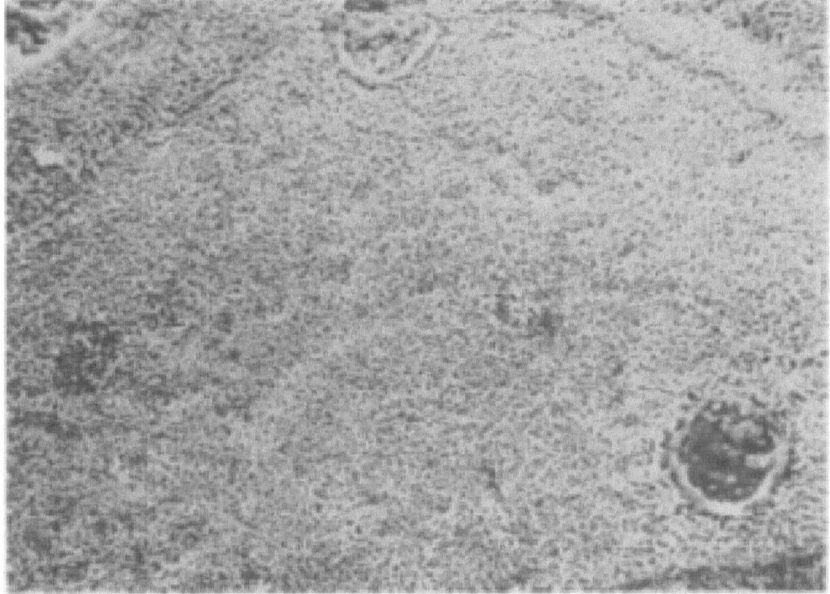

Fig. II-8. — Appearance of the microvilli and craters on the surface of normal rabbit cornea. Scanning electron microscopy. × 6560.

metabolism. This correlates well with histochemical and biochemical studies. The epithelium contains high activity of enzymes of glycolysis, Kreb's cycle and Na^+ and K^+ activated ATPase. Glycogen, glutathione and abscorbic acid are also present. Although acetylcholine and cholinestrases are present in high concentrations, their function in corneal epithelium is unknown. They may play a role in cation transport or trophic nerve function.

In contrast to this high enzymatic activity, ultrastructural studies of the corneal epithelium have shown the paucity of cell organelles. Small mitochondria are present in the basal cells and the deeper layers of the wing cells. Cytoplasmic filaments are more pronounced in the superficial cells, almost completely obscuring the cellular organisation.

On the surface the cell membranes form a large number of finger-like projections about 0.2μ in length, best seen by scanning electron microscopy (fig. II-8). These are called microvilli. In well prepared specimens studied by transmission electron microscopy, the mucoid material from tear film may be seen sticking to them.

The number of microvilli varies. Some cells are devoid of micro-villi, and appear dark under the scanning electron microscope. They show other degenerative changes, i.e. fragmented or incomplete nuclei and disappearance of a part of the cytoplasm. They are desquamating cells. Their desmosomal attachments may be ruptured. There are also "intermediate" cells having the appearence between the normal and desquamating cells.

It has been estimated that the corneal epithelium is constantly renewed every 7 days. Employing the tritium labelled thymidine incorporation, Hanna and O'Brien (1960) found that the basal epithe-lial cells moved out to be sloughed off the superficial layer within $3\frac{1}{2}$ to 7 days.

Terminal branches of the nerves are found among the basal cells of the epithelium. In the corneal stroma all nerves are surrounded by Schwann cells. At the lavel of the basement membrane the nerve endings lose their accompanying Schwann cells and become embed-ded in the basal or lateral wall of the epithelial cells.

Basement membrane

This membrane is 0.75 to 1.5 μ thick (fig. II-7). According to Jakus (1961) it consists of very fine tightly packed filaments, but Kayes and Holmberg (1960) and Teng (1961) could not recognise any distinct fibers. This membrane is thicker and more electron dense at the desmosomes than between them. Many small projections from the posterior surface of the basement membrane into the Bowman's layer maintain a firm bond between both layers. Histochemically, the basement membrane contains lipids, polysaccharides and reticular fibers.

Bowman's layer

Bowman's layer separates the epithelial basement membrane from stroma. This layer is present only in primates and man. It varies from 8 to 14 μ in thickness and appears structureless by light micros-copy. Under electron microscope it shows many fine non-oriented collagen fibers lying in structureless electron dense material (fig. II-7). The Bowman's layer is acellular.

The posterior border of the Bowman's layer is indistinct. Its unoriented fibers enter between the well oriented stromal fibers. It does not differ from corneal stroma in histochemical reactions.

Stroma

Underlying the Bowman's layer are well organised bundles of collagen fibers called lamellae. The bundles interlace with each other but generally remain parallel to the surface. The collagen fibers are embedded in a ground substance composed of mucopolysaccharides. The perfect optical transparency of the cornea is still somewhat of a mystery. One would expect that the mixture of collagen fibers of a rather high refractive index of 1.555, and mucopolysaccharide medium of refractive index 1.345, would produce a white opalescent tissue such as sclera. According to the hypothesis of Maurice (1957) the transparency is due to the regular spacing of the collagen fibers.

This hypothesis explains very well why the deformation of the cornea, for example during surgical manipulations, produces instant cloudiness which disappears immediately when the deformation ceases.

The hypothesis also explains how a slight excess of hydration produces a marked turbidity by disturbing the regular pattern of the collagen fibers. The fact that it has been impossible to observe the regular pattern in fixed corneal preparations is not a valid objection against Maurice's hypothesis. Every known fixation method spoils the transparency of the cornea during its processing.

The flattened cell bodies of keratocytes are seen between the collagen fibers. In normal corneas they contain scanty cytoplasm and cell organelles but well defined nuclei. Different keratocytes may establish contact with one another by long cytoplasmic processes which extend between the collagen bundles.

Descemet's membrane

This very elastic structureless membrane bounds the posterior surface of the stroma. It is about 10 µ thick.

According to Jakus (1961) it is made of collagen-like material which does not show a high degree of organization. It is rich in glycine and hydroxyproline. Glycoproteins are bound to the protein moiety. Descemet's membrane stains intensely with PAS. It is considered to be the product of secretion of endothelial cells.

Endothelium

The corneal endothelium consists of a single layer of flat hexagonal cells lining the posterior surface of Descemet's membrane. The lateral surfaces of the cells are convoluted and the nuclei are regularly spaced. In comparison to the epithelial cells the endothelial cells contain relatively large number of mitochondria, vesicles and granules. The cytoplasmic tonofilaments as seen in the epithelial cells are lacking. The desmosomes are also absent.

The endothelial cell population decreases with age. The morphology of cells can be evaluated in vivo by specular microscopy.

Endothelium plays an important role in the electrolyte transfer into and out of the cornea; and hence in the maintenance of its state of deturgescence.

BIBLIOGRAPHY

Cotlier, E. — The cornea. In: *Adler's physiology of the eye, clinical application.* Ed. Moses R. A., Mosby Co, St. Louis, 1975.

Delmarcelle, Y., François, J., Goes, F., Collignon-Brach, J. et Verbraeken, H. — Biométrie oculaire clinique (oculométrie). *Bull. Soc. belge d'Ophtal., 172,* 1, 1976.

Gipson, I. K. and Anderson, R. A. — Actin filaments in normal and migrating corneal epithelial cells. *Invest. Ophthal. Vis. Sci., 16,* 161, 1977.

Hanna, C. and O'Brien, J. E. — Cell production and migration in the epithelial layer of the cornea. *Arch. Ophthal., 64,* 536, 1960.

Jakus, M. A. — The fine structure of the human cornea. In: *The structure of the eye.* Ed. Smelser, G. K., Academic Press. N.Y. 1961.

Kayes, J. and Holmberg, A. — The fine structure of Bowman's layer and the basement membrane of the corneal epithelium. *Amer. J. Ophthal., 50,* 1013, 1960.

Maudgal, P. C. — The epithelial response in keratitis sicca and keratitis herpetica (an experimental and clinical study). Doctoral Thesis. University of Leuven, 1976. *Doc. Ophthal., 45,* 223, 1978.

Maudgal, P. C. and Missotten, L. — Histology and histochemistry of the normal superficial corneal epithelium of rabbit. *Alb. v. Graefes Arch. Klin. expt. Ophthal., 205,* 167, 1978.

Maurice, D. M. — The structure and transparency of the cornea. *J. Physiol. (London), 136,* 263, 1957.

Missotten, L. and Maudgal, P. C. — The replica technique used to study superficial corneal epithelium in vivo. *Amer. J. Ophthal., 84,* 104, 1977.

Prijot, E., Weekers, R. et Marechal, C. — Variations topographiques du rayon de courbure de la cornée. Son importance pour la prescription des lentilles cornéennes. *Bull. Soc. belge d'Ophtal., 138,* 429, 1964.

Rahi, A. and Ashton, N. — Contractile proteins in retinal endothelium and other non-muscle tissues of the eye. *Brit. J. Ophthal., 62,* 627, 1978.

Teng, C. C. — The fine structure of the corneal epithelium and basement membrane of the rabbit. *Amer. J. Ophthal., 51,* 278, 1961.

CHAPTER III

HEALING OF THE EPITHELIUM

Earlier studies of corneal epithelium healing have been discussed in detail by Duke-Elder and Leigh (1965) and recently reviewed by Lemp (1976). The epithelial repair involves two distinct processes. The epithelial defect is first covered by sliding of the surrounding epithelial cells (fig. III-1) accompanied by temporary cessation of mitotic activity and exfoliation. After a latent period mitotic activity increases resulting in the thickening of epithelial layer. A variable number of polymorphonuclear leukocytes appear at the wound edge after 3 hours. They originate from the conjunctival capillaries and in the case of a central corneal wound travel solely through the tear film (Robb and Kuwabara, 1962). The leukocytes are attracted probably by the release of chemotactic substances due to tissue injury, as no microbial agents have been detected in these studies. The polymorphonuclear leukocytes do not disappear until after the wound is covered by the sliding epithelium.

Sliding of cells

The phenomenon of epithelial sliding has been investigated by different techniques and in different types of corneal injury. Pfister (1975) studied 6 mm corneal erosions of rabbits by scanning electron microscopy. Five minutes after an abrasion the epithelial cells within 0.5 to 1 mm of the defect become retracted and appear to detach from one another. The tight interdigitations between adjacent cells disappear, but the desmosomes are not ruptured and the cells retain some contact with the neighboring cells (Kuwabara et al., 1976).

The surface microvilli are lost. The epithelial migration begins one hour after injury (Friedenwald and Buschke, 1944) and has been noted to reach the bottom of the wound crater in 4 to 12 hours (Robb and Kuwabara, 1962; Hanna, 1966; Bracher, 1967; Matsuda and Smelser, 1973; and Kuwabara et al., 1976) depending on the size of the wound and its depth.

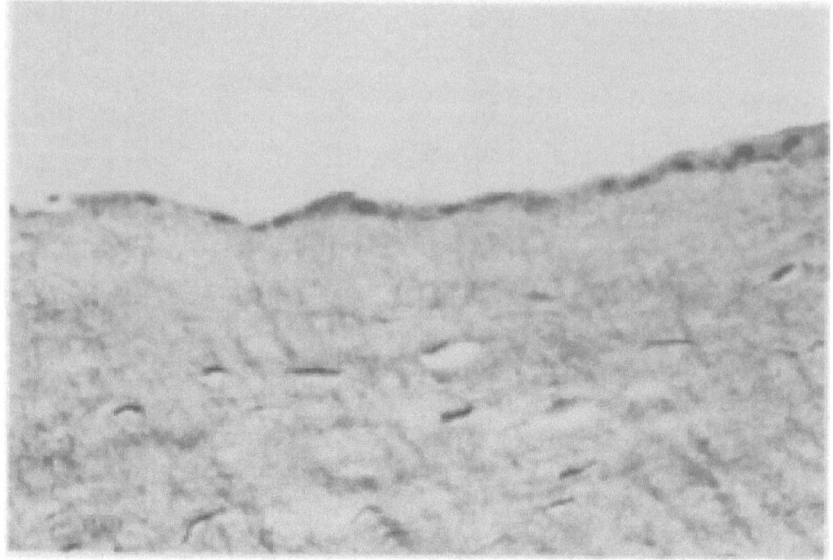

Fig. III-1. — Healing of epithelium 1 day after a corneal replica. One layer of cells migrated to cover the defects. H.E. × 375.

In contrast to the opinion of earlier authors (Friedenwald and Buschke, 1944), Hanna (1966) by thymidine-H^3 tagging of cells, conclusively demonstrated that all the cell layers participate in sliding. According to Kuwabara et al. (1976), the cells of the basal layer slide to a lesser extent. The main sliding cells are the wing cells, but the flat superficial cells regain the cytoplasmic constituents of the younger cells and slide similarly.

In our studies on the response of corneal epithelium to blunt trauma (unpublished), we found marked transformation of superficial cells adjacent to the wounded area (figs. III-2 and III-3). At the edge of abrasion the epithelial cells become flattened. The flattened and expanded portions of the cells are devoid of microvilli (Pfister, 1975). After six hours ruffling of cell surface appears in some cells. The ruffles are thin elevations of cell membrane and may be the first sign of cell movement.

Gipson and Anderson (1977), for the first time, demonstrated the presence of actin filaments along the basal membrane of the sliding cells at their advancing edges and in the cytoplasmic processes. In normal circumstances the actin filaments were seen only along the superficial plasma membranes of the superficial cells. It is likely that

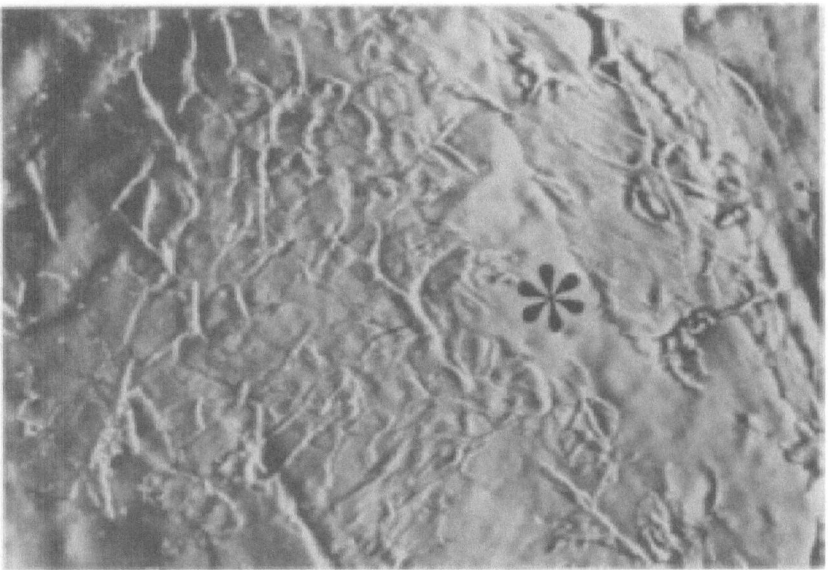

Fig. III-2. — Superficial cells have become retracted adjacent to the traumatic area (∗). Corneal replica was made 20 minutes after experimental trauma. Oblique illumination microscopy. × 135.

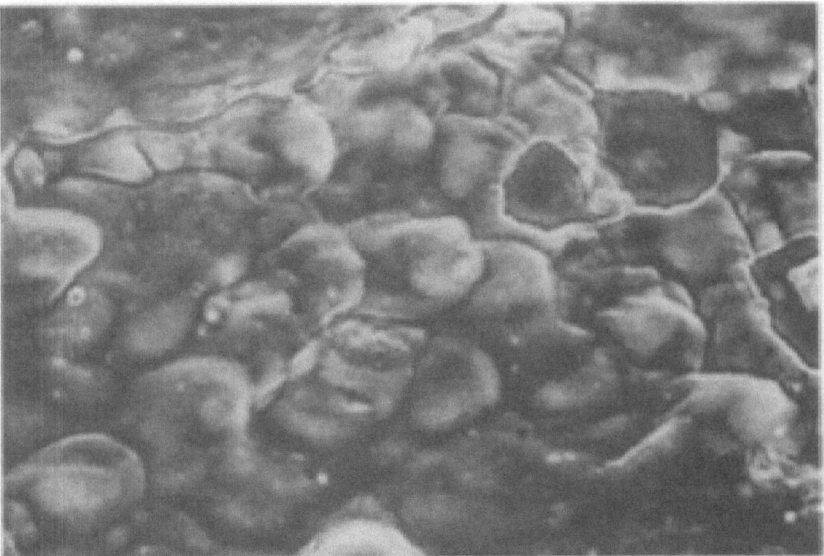

Fig. III-3. — Appearance of the traumatic area 2 hours after blunt trauma. The epithelial cells appear rounded. Phase contrast microscopy of the replica. × 213.

the ruffles are produced by the contractile activity of these filaments.

The ruffles vary widely in thickness and length. From the thicker ruffles large tongue-like processes extend out of the cells to touch the denuded surface of the cornea. These cytoplasmic extensions are called pseudopodia or filopodia.

The filopodia also vary in length and thickness. Occasionally upto 100μ long cytoplasmic processes extend from the cells at the wound margin onto the denuded stroma and terminate in a pad of cytoplasm (Pfister, 1975). The filopodia formation occurs only along the advancing edge of the cells. Two adjacent cells often touch one another by ruffles and filopodia. In the case of overlapping only the top cell shows ruffling and filopodia. A second or third layer of cells may advance over the first and second layer respectively. The migrating epithelial cells never become free from the surrounding cells. New desmosomes are formed where the cytoplasmic extensions come in contact (Kuwabara et al., 1976). The sliding cells maintain the normal cytological structure except the disappearance of glycogen granules. However, the cytoplasmic activity of glycolytic enzymes remains normal.

In deep non-perforating wounds of the cornea (Kuwabara et al, 1976), the epithelial cells that come to rest at the base of defect increase in height in 24 hours and begin to regain the characteristics of basal cells. The adjacent cells interdigitate with each other but up to 24 hours a linear space may be seen along the opposing surfaces of the epithelial cells of the wound edges.

In penetrating wounds (Matsuda and Smelser, 1973) the corneal wound is first plugged in its posterior part by a fibrinous exudate which is covered by sliding epithelium. The rest of the healing process is similar to non-penetrating wounds.

The ruffling and filopodial activity continues till the denuded area is completely covered by epithelium. In the studies of Pfister (1975) a 0.5 mm residual defect was left after 38 hours. After 55 hours there was no residual defect but the surface cells appeared darker due to the lack of microvilli. After 114 hours the corneal surface was normal by scanning electron microscopy.

The epithelial sliding in wound healing is an orderly phenomenon, but the factors controlling the cell movement are not well understood. In full thickness explants of rabbit cornea grown in a tissue culture medium, the cell migration stopped when the sliding epithelial cells came in contact with the endothelial cells. However, if the endothelium was removed from the explants beforehand, the migration of epithelial cells continued to cover the explant on all sides (Cameron et al., 1974). The phenomenon of cell movement inhibition after contact with other cells is called "contact inhibition". Martz and Steinberg (1973) proposed several theories of contact inhibition, but the exact mechanism is unknown. Johnson et al. (1972) showed that an increase in the cyclic AMP concentration in the fibroblast cultures inhibited cell migration. The authors concluded that contact between the two cell surfaces may result in the generation of such a substance as a signal for inhibition. However, the phenomenon of contact inhibition for the same type of cells can be modified by changing environmental factors in tissue cultures (Cameron et al., 1974; Yanoff, 1976).

Sliding of the epithelium requires energy which may be derived from the cellular glycogen. If glycogen is extracted with a weak amylase solution before incubation (Kuwabara et al., 1976), sliding of the epithelium is extremely retarded and the cells undergo degeneration. The sliding is reactivated in glucose rich medium. The sliding cells show a high lactic acid dehydrogenase activity.

Metabolic poisons, such as parhydroxymercuribenzoate (10^{-6} M) and iodo-acetic acid (10^{-5} M) inhibit sliding (Kuwabara et al., 1976). In the studies of the same authors variation of pH from 6 to 8 or modification of the atmospheric gases i.e. oxygen, nitrogen and carbon dioxide, did not influence the cell movement of cultured rabbit corneal epithelium. No sliding of epithelium was observed above 42 °C and below 4 °C. Between 24 and 38 °C only slight enhancement of sliding was noted. Epithelial sliding is also inhibited by systemic administration of morphine, high doses of ephedrine and epinephrine and local application of anesthetics. Superior cervical ganglionectomy does not affect the sliding process (Friedenwald and Buschke, 1944).

During healing the corneal epithelium produces collagenase, if the wound extends to the stroma (Brown and Weller, 1970). The physiological role of the enzyme in wound healing may be the production of collagen precursors to be presented to the corneal fibroblasts. It might also act as a monitor and prevent excessive collagen synthesis in the healing wound.

Davanger and Evensen (1971) presented evidence that the limbal palisades of Vogt may be the site of epithelial regeneration, assuming that the basal cell population of the normal corneal epithelium could be an insufficient source to supply the cells to cover the entire denuded cornea. In contrast to the basal epithelial cells of cornea, the limbal palisades consist of richly vascularised subepithelial papillae, between which the ridgelike radial thickenings of the epithelium project downwards.

In coloured people paired radial pigmented lines are seen between the palisades which may be due to the presence of melanin in basal cells. In guinea pig experiments pigment migration was seen to follow the epithelial cell growth over the corneal defect. The limbal pigment became lighter in the corresponding area. After 5 days the corneal pigment disappeared and the limbal pigment became normal.

After total removal of the corneal epithelium, conjunctival epithelium migrates over the cornea (Duke Elder and Leigh, 1965). Initially, the regenerating epithelium over cornea shows the characteristics of the conjunctival epithelium, i.e. presence of goblet cells and an irregular thick structure. After 2 to 3 weeks the cells gradually attain the characteristics of corneal epithelium. Although the histological transformation of epithelium of conjunctival origin in rabbits may be completed within 6 weeks after corneal abrasions produced by scraping or iodine cautery, the biochemical transformation is not; especially in the chemically damaged corneas (Thoft and Friend, 1977). Also the healing rate of conjunctivally derived epithelium is slower (Friend and Thoft, 1978), perhaps due to the lack of glycogen in these cells.

Mitosis

The thickening of the epithelial layers, after the wound is covered by sliding cells, is achieved by the proliferation of the cells by mitotic division. Having labelled the cells with thymidine-H^3, Hanna (1966) showed that immediately after the injury the DNA synthesis in the epithelial cells markedly decreased in a zone extending about 120 epithelial cell lengths from the wound edge. Beyond this zone of decreased thymidine-H^3 uptake a narrow band of basal cells showed marked increase in thymidine uptake and mitosis after 24 hours. This zone of mitosis shifted to the center of the wound in 3 to 6 days, depending on the size of the wound crater. Similar findings were reported by Kuwabara et al (1976) in their ultrastructural study.

There was no difference in the pattern of thymidine H^3 incorporation and mitosis in the healing of penetrating and non-penetrating wounds. In superficial corneal burns in rats, if only the superficial cells were killed, the adjacent basal epithelial cells showed increased thymidine-H^3 incorporation between 8 and 24 hours. The zone of decreased thymidine-H^3 uptake was absent.

Epithelial regeneration in large thermal burns of the cornea is achieved almost exclusively by mitosis (Duke Elder and Leigh, 1965).

Ultraviolet light exposure of 10 seconds or less increases the rate of mitosis whereas X-radiation has the opposite effect (in rats). Longer exposures to U.V. light, metabolic poisons and anoxia inhibit mitosis. (Duke Elder and Leigh, 1965; Kuwabara et al., 1976; Lemp, 1976.)

Recently the epidermal growth factor (EGF) isolated from mice submaxillary glands (Ho et al. 1974) and fibroblast growth factor, isolated from bovine pituitary glands and bovine brains (Gospodaro-wicz et al., 1977) have been shown to promote healing due to their mitogenic effect on the corneal epithelium in vivo and in organ culture. No toxic effects of EGF were observed on the rabbit corneas with or without intact epithelium. However, immunogenic reactions of this polypeptide may interfere with its therapeutic application in man.

Regeneration of basement membrane

Basement membrane plays an important role in the adhesion of epithelium to cornea. In corneal abrasions, where the basement membrane is left intact, a firm adhesion of regenerated epithelium occurs in about five days (Khodadoust, 1967).

However, no morphological changes have been detected at the level of the basement membrane or in the basal epithelial cells which could explain this increased adhesion (Khodadoust et al., 1968). In rabbits after superficial lamellar keratectomy, adhesion of epithelium was absent, upto about six weeks after operation, until a new basement membrane had regenerated.

Using electron microscopic and immunological techniques, the intracellular origin of epithelial basement membrane has been demonstrated (Andres et al., 1962; Kurtz and Feldman, 1962; Pierce et al., 1964). After keratectomy, the regeneration of basement membrane does not begin untill the wound is covered by epithelium and the cell movement has stopped (Kenyon, 1969; Blümke et al., 1969). The morphological changes leading to the synthesis of basement membrane are interpreted in different ways by these authors.

Kenyon (1969) noticed the perinuclear vesicles containing basement membrane-like material, and basement membrane lined infoldings of the basal cell plasma membrane in contact with stroma, after 7 days of post operative regeneration. By gradual eversion of these basement membrane lined infoldings the basement membrane comes to lie on the flat lower surface of the basal cells. In this way, synthesis of discrete lengths of basement membrane material, piece by piece, may restore the continuous basement membrane. According to Blümcke et al. (1969), the regeneration of the basement membrane first involves the accumulation of tufts of filamentous structures, about 30 Å wide, on the internal side of the plasma membrane. The tufts of filaments pierce the plasma membrane and might connect with the similar structures forming an irregular network outside the cell, which later differentiates into two discrete layers, a very thin and discontinuous near the plasma membrane and a thick basement membrane proper, parallel and below it. Eventually, the tufts may develop into the special points of attachment i.e. hemidesmosomes.

In summary, an epithelial defect is repaired first by sliding of epithelial cells, an active process requiring glycogen, mediated by actin fibers and inhibited by some metabolic poisons and local anesthetics. The normal thickness of the epithelium is restored by mitosis. The basement membrane is necessary for a firm adhesion of the regenerated epithelium.

BIBLIOGRAPHY

Andres, G. A., Morgan, C., Hsu, K. C., Rifkind, R. A. and Seegal, B. C. — The basement membranes and cisternae of visceral epithelium cells in nephritic rat glomeruli. *J. Exp. Med.*, *115*, 929, 1962.
Blümcke, S., Rode, J. and Niedorf, H. R. — Formation of the basement membrane during regeneration of the corneal epithelium. *Z. Zellforsch.*, *93*, 84, 1969.
Bracher, R. — Radioautographic analysis of the synthesis of protein, RNA, DNA, and sulphated mucopolysaccharides in the early stages of corneal wound healing. Invest. Ophthal., *6*, 565, 1967.
Brown, S. I., and Weller, C. A. — Cell origin of collagenase in normal and wounded corneas. *Arch. Ophthal.*, *83*, 74, 1970.
Cameron, J. D., Flayman, B. A. and Yanoff, M. — In vitro studies of corneal wound healing: epithelial-endothelial interactions. *Invest. Ophthal.*, *13*, 575, 1974.

Davanger, M. and Evensen, A. — Role of the pericorneal papillary structure in renewal of corneal epithelium. *Nature, 229,* 560, 1971.

Duke-Elder, S. and Leigh, A. G. — System of Ophthalmology, Vol. VIII. Diseases of the outer eye. Duke-Elder S. (Ed.), Henry Kimpton, London, 1965.

Friedenwald, J. S. and Buschke, W. — Influence of some experimental variables on the epithelial movements in the healing of corneal wounds. *J. Cell. Comp. Physiol., 23,* 95, 1944.

Friend, J. and Thoft, R. A. — Functional competence of regenerating ocular surface epithelium. *Invest. Ophthal. Vis. Sci., 17,* 134, 1978.

Gipson, I. K. and Anderson, R. A. — Actin filaments in normal and migrating corneal epithelial cells. *Invest. Ophthal. Vis. Sci., 16,* 161, 1977..

Gospodarowicz, D., Mescher, A. L., Brown, K. D. and Birdwell, C. R. — The role of fibroblast growth factor and epidermal growth factor in the proliferative response of the corneal and lens epithelium. *Exp. Eye Res., 25,* 631, 1977.

Hanna, C. and O'Brien, J. E. — Cell production and migration in the epithelial layer of the cornea. *Arch. Ophthal., 64,* 536, 1960.

Hanna, C. — Proliferation and migration of epithelial cells. *Amer. J. Ophthal., 61,* 55, 1966.

Ho, P. D., Davis, W. H., Elliott, J. H and Cohen, S. — Kinetics of corneal epithelial regeneration and epidermal growth factor. *Invest. Ophthal., 13,* 804, 1974.

Johnson, G. S., Morgan, W. D. and Pastan, I. — Regulation of cell motility by cyclic AMP, *Nature, 235,* 54, 1972.

Kenyon, K. R. — The synthesis of basement membrane by the corneal epithelium in bullous keratopathy. *Invest. Ophthal., 8,* 156, 1969.

Khodadoust, A. A. — Techniques for the preparation of sheets of pure corneal epithelium. *Amer. J. Ophthal., 63,* 942, 1967.

Khodadoust, A. A., Silverstein, A. M., Kenyon, K. R. and Dowling, J. E. — Adhesion of regenerating corneal epithelium. *Amer. J. Ophthal., 65,* 339, 1968.

Kurtz, S. M. and Feldman, J. D. — Experimental studies on the formation of glomerular basement membrane *J. Ultrastruct. Res., 6,* 19, 1962.

Kuwabara, J., Perkins, D. G. and Cogan, D. G. — Sliding of the epithelium in experimental corneal wounds. *Invest. Ophthal., 15,* 4, 1976.

Lemp, M. A. — Cornea and sclera. *Arch. Ophthal., 94,* 473, 1976.

Martz, E. and Steinberg, M. S. — Contact inhibition of what? An analytical review. *J. Cell. Physiol., 81,* 25, 1973.

Matsuda, H. and Smelser, G. K. — Electron microscopy of corneal wound healing. *Exp. Eye Res., 16,* 427, 1973.

Pfister, R. R. — The healing of corneal epithelial abrasions in the rabbit: A scanning electron microscope study. *Invest. Ophthal., 14,* 648, 1975.

Pierce, G. B., Beals, T. F., Sriram, J. S. and Midgley, A. R. — Basement membrane IV. Epithelial origin and immunologic cross reactions. *Amer. J. Path., 45,* 929, 1964.

Robb, R. M. and Kuwabara, J. — Corneal wound healing I. The movement of polymorphonuclear leukocytes into corneal wounds. *Arch. Ophthal., 68,* 636, 1962.

Thoft, R. A. and Friend, J. — Biochemical transformation of regenerating ocular surface epithelium. *Invest. Ophthal. Vis. Sci., 17,* 134, 1977.

Yanoff, M. — Biology in vitro of corneal epithelium and endothelium. *Documenta Ophthal., 41,* 157, 1976.

CHAPTER IV

CORNEAL EROSIONS

Erosions of the cornea are very common, occurring in a wide variety of corneal diseases. They may occur as multiple punctate lesions or as recurrent erosions and persistent aseptic defects of the epithelium. The last two entites together are sometimes termed *epithelial erosion syndrome*.

Multiple punctate erosions

Premature desquamation of superficial epithelial cells produces multiple punctate erosions. Exposure of the underlying immature cells causes pain and irritation accompanied by lacrimation and photophobia. Clinically the erosions appear as very fine, slightly depressed spots, localized to a small part or dispersed all over cornea. Sometimes they become visible only after fluorescein staining. Treatment of multiple erosions depends on the underlying etiological factor (table IV-1).

Recurrent erosions

Recurrent corneal erosions are solitary or multiple gross epithelial defects characteristically recurring repeatedly over an interval of weeks or months, spontaneously or after apparent healing of a traumatic corneal abrasion (Duke-Elder and Leigh, 1965).

Etiological considerations

Hansen (1877), first drew attention to recurrent erosions. v. Szily sen. (1900) and Franke (1906) observed traumatic as well as non traumatic spontaneously occurring recurrent corneal erosions. Hirtsch (1898), Salus (1922), Proksch (1926), Specktor (1931) and more recently Tripathi and Bron (1972) described spontaneously occurring bilateral corneal erosions. However, in other cases bilateral involvement may follow corneal trauma (Flynn and Esterly, 1966). France-

TABLE IV-1. — *Disease conditions causing multiple punctate erosions*

A. *Mechanical*
   Abrasive dusts
   Foreign bodies
   Trichiasis
   Palpebral vernal conjunctivitis

B. *Chemical*
   Mustard gas keratitis
   Artificial silk keratitis

C. *Toxic*
   Warts and molluscum bodies of lids

D. *Infective*
   a. Bacterial infections
      Various forms of bacterial keratoconjunctivitis
      Staphylococcal blepharoconjunctivitis
      (Seborrhaeic blepharitis)
   b. Viral infections:
      Trachoma
      Inclusion conjunctivitis
      Lymphogranuloma venerium
      Herpes simplex
      Herpes zoster
      Vaccinia

E. *Dry eyes*
   Sjögren's syndrome
   Reiter's disease
   Erythema multiforme
   Benign mucus membrane pemphigoid
   Ichtyosis
   Ocular pemphigoid
   Steven-Johnson syndrome

F. *Irradiational*
   Undue exposure to X-rays; β and γ-rays and U.V. light

schetti (1928) showed autosomal dominant inheritance of recurrent erosions in a family. In 1958 when this familial study was braught upto date, a total of 40 members over 6 generations had suffered from this disease. (Franceschetti and Klein, 1961). Wales (1955) reported a similar type of inheritance in a family.

Occasionally, recurrent erosions may form the presenting symptom of corneal dystrophies i.e. lattice like (Duke-Elder and Leigh, 1965; Valle, 1967), or the macular forms (Franceschetti and Klein, 1961; Duke-Elder and Leigh, 1965; and Valle, 1967). Rarely, recurrent corneal erosions may occur in the healthy members of a family showing parenchymatous corneal degeneration (Hermann, 1946). Gifford (1925) drew attention to the occurrence of recurrent erosions in Fuchs' dystrophy. One of his patients suffered from recurrent erosions in one eye and Fuchs' endothelial dystrophy in the fellow eye.

Valle (1967) studied 30 members of a family over 3 generations. One member suffered from Fuchs' dystrophy. In the next two generations recurrent erosions developed in 6 members, whereas the children of the healthy siblings were unaffected. Recurrent erosions have also been described in association with map-dot-fingerprint dystrophy, Meesmans' dystrophy, and Reis-Buckler's dystrophy (Trobe and Laibson, 1972; Bron and Triphathi, 1973; Tripathi and Bron, 1973; Rodrigues and Laibson, 1976). In addition to these rather infrequent cases of recurrent erosion in association with corneal dystrophies we see numerous patients with typical recurrent erosions due to trauma. In our experience recurrent corneal erosions are more prone to develop after a lacerating or macerating corneal abrasion with non-sterile objects like twigs, tree branches, plant leaves, finger nails, screw drivers, etc., rather than a relatively clean wound of an iron foreignbody. The initial corneal trauma may have been so trivial that the patient forgets about it altogether at the time of acute episode. However, history of previous trauma can usually be elicited on questioning.

Sturrock (1976) presented evidence that recurrent erosions may develop due to nocturnal lagophthalmos.

Clinical picture

Typically, the patient wakes up in the morning with an acutely painful eye with foreign body sensation, lacrimation and photophobia. The symptoms are so characteristic that some patients are afraid to open their eyes on waking-up. In other cases the patient may be aroused from sleep in the night by sharp pain.

The upper eyelid is somewhat swollen. The eye is moderately red. Biomicroscopy reveals circumcorneal injection. The corneal epithelium may be raised at the site of lesion containing rounded swollen cells and intraepithelial microcysts. Exfoliation of these cells leads to an epithelial defect. Irrespective of the initial site of injury, in posttraumatic cases, the recurrent corneal erosion is generally located midway between the limbus and lower pupillary margin (fig. IV-1). The horizontally elongated lesion has tapering ends which do not involve the limbal area. Fluorescein staining may demonstrate multiple areas of cell exfoliation in the lesion. Also, fluorescein diffuses into the lesion, staining the loosely attached surrounding epithelium (fig. IV-2). There is minimal edema of the subepithelial stroma and a minimal infiltration by wandering cells.

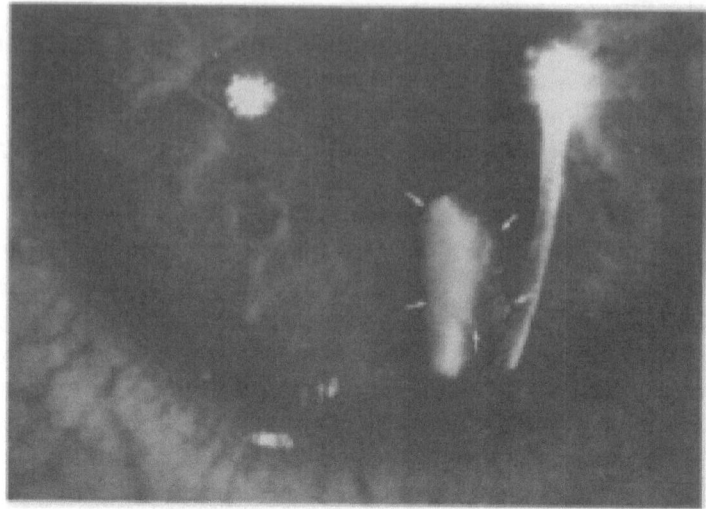

Fig. IV-1. — Post-traumatic recurrent corneal erosion (arrows) observed in retro-illumination.

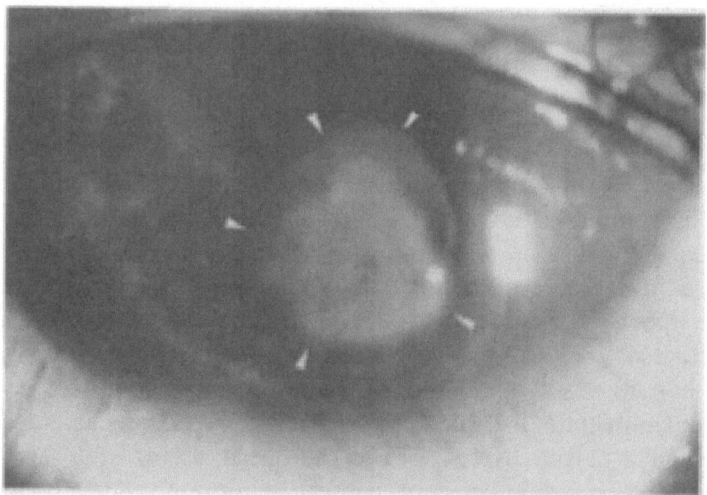

Fig. IV-2. — Fluorescein diffuses rapidly into the areas of loosely attached epithelium (arrows) surrounding a recurrent erosion.

In the cases of spontaneous erosions and those occuring in corneal dystrophies, the erosions may be multiple but vary in size and shape. Unfortunately, they have predilection for central cornea in which case the vision is markedly affected.

The corneal sensitivity is generally normal but may be reduced.

Small lesions may heal spontaneously in one hour or two days at the most, but the larger ones continue to cause distress if unattended. Between the acute episodes the cornea may show small subepithelial greyish spots, with or without microcysts, at the site of healed erosions. Recurrences occur invariably in the same area.

Histopathology

Earlier investigators did not find anything specific in their histopathological sudies (Duke-Elder and Leigh, 1965). The epithelium changes included intra- and extracellular edema with vesicle formation and necrosis. These findings have been confirmed in recent histological and ultrastructural studies. Goldmann et al. (1969), in addition, found some flattened cells in the basal layer of the epithelium and areas of defective basement membrane. Hemidesmosomes were absent or poorly developed in these areas. Tripathi and Bron (1972 and 1973) confirmed the absence or degeneration of basement membrane but noted groups of poorly staining "pale cells," by light

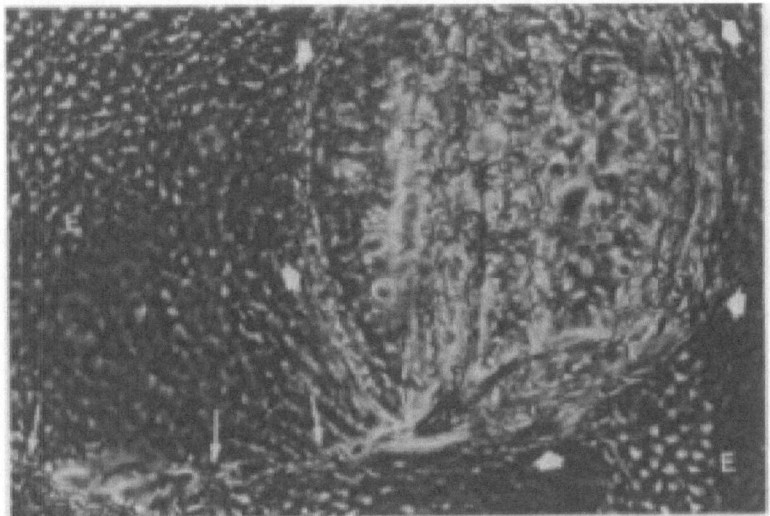

Fig. IV-3. — Corneal replica of a post-traumatic recurrent erosion. The area of large erosion (broad arrows) contains some rounded and swollen cells surrounded by edematous epithelium (E). Small arrows indicate a healing area along a linear line. Phase contrast microscopy. × 120.

and electron microscopy, in a case of spontaneous bilateral recurrent erosion. They also observed intraepithelial microcysts containing some PAS positive material and degenerated epithelial cells. Similar cysts are found in other epithelial dystrophies (Tripathi and Bron, 1973; Polack, 1976). Preliminary studies by corneal replicas demonstrate irregularly arranged swollen epithelium cells in the area of erosion. The elongated epithelial cells typically bordering the dendritic ulcers (Maudgal and Missotten, 1978) are absent in recurrent erosions (fig. IV-3).

Pathogenesis

Pathogenesis of this condition is still unknown. Although we know that the basement membrane plays an important role in the attachment of epithelium to the cornea (Khodadoust, 1967; Khodadoust et al., 1968), yet it remains disputable if its defect in the recurrent erosions is the primary lesion resulting in epithelial changes, or secondary to some abnormality in the epithelial cells. The basement membrane is secreted by the basal epithelium cells. Even in the edematous states, epithelial cells attempt to repair the basement membrane (Kenyon, 1969). Such a repair process has not been demonstrated in recurrent erosions. It implies that the primary defect may lie in the epithelium itself. Duke-Elder and Leigh (1965) suggested that the epithelium may be dystrophic in nature and the corneal injury may act only as a trigger mechanism. This speculation is supported by occasional bilateral spontaneous recurrence of corneal erosions and that in corneal dystrophies. Also, the chances of healing are much better if the loosely attached epithelium is rubbed away with a cotton tipped applicator, or after chemical cauterization (Duke-Elder and Leigh, 1965) and the corneal replica procedure (Maudgal and Missotten, in preparation). All these methods destroy the loosely attached epithelium which allows an entirely new epithelium to regenerate. If the primary defect was in the basement membrane, healing should not take place after such procedures.

Sturrock (1976) collected 102 patients presenting with the signs and symptoms of corneal erosions after sleeping with open eyes. Forty nine patients had had multiple attacks but bilateral corneal changes were seen only in 18 cases. In some cases the attacks occurred on several mornings in succession. The author also concluded from literature that Bell's phenomenon (the eyes turn up during sleep, thus protecting the corneas from dehydration during exposure) was not consistent in all subjects and could be present one night and absent the next, or vice versa. Nocturnal lagophthalmos may also not be a bilateral or constant phenomenon. This could explain the occurrence of acute episodes in succession, or at variable intervals, when the nocturnal lagophthalmos is accompanied by the absence of Bell's phenomenon. If is difficult to ascertain if nocturnal lagophthalmos and corneal exposure are operative in all cases of recurrent erosions. It is equally unknown if the corneal epithelium of post-traumatic eyes is more sensitive to such an exposure than normal eyes; as we regularly see only a punctate staining of lower cornea in patients with nocturnal lagophthalmos. However, if the above mentioned phenomenon constitutes an etiological factor of recurrent erosions, it could explain their typical location.

Treatment

The treatment of a recurrent corneal erosion (Duke-Elder and Leigh, 1965) constitutes the application of antibiotics to prevent secondary infection, instillation of cycloplegics to overcome ciliary spasm and a firmly applied bandage to prevent lid movement, which could mechanically tear-away the regenerating epithelium. A soft corneal or scleral contact lens may also be fitted to protect the cornea from rubbing action of lids. Removal of loosely attached epithelium around an erosion by a cotton-tipped applicator, leaving a clean circumscribed margin, or its destruction by chemical cauterization using carbolic acid, 10% trichloractic acid, 20% zinc sulphate or iodo-alcohol, have been reported to be effective. We have treated all types of erosions by the corneal replica procedure with considerable success. In resistant cases lamellar keratoplasty may be effective (Duke-Elder and Leigh, 1965).

To prevent the recurrences of acute episodes (Duke-Elder and Leigh, 1965) instillation of an emolient or lubricant is widely advocated. By lubricating the eye, this prevents the possible mechanical effect of the lids on waking up. Use of emolients would also protect the cornea from damage due to lagophthalmos. However, methylcellulose, if used as a lubricant, is sticky and therefore annoying. We prescribe nightly application of lanolin and mineral oil ointment in white petrolatum (Duratears®) which is not sticky and well tolerated. Use of a thin soft contact lens may achieve the same purpose. To reduce epithelial edema, which may arise due to the lack of tear evaporation during sleep; application of hyperosmotic agents before sleep is advised by some authors (Trobe and Laibson, 1972; Krachmer, 1974). Despite treatment, some cases show repeated breakdown of the epithelium and develop persistent epithelial defects.

Persistent aseptic epithelial defects

Aseptic epithelial defects differ from recurrent erosions in being larger, persistent and remain denuded of epithelium despite treatment. If the regeneration of epithelium takes place, it soon breaks down. The classification of etiological factors in persistent epithelium defects is given in table IV-2. Aseptic epithelial defects may develop after severe corneal insults like chemical and thermal burns, corneal denervation, surgical trauma, metaherpetic keratitis and degenerative or edematous states of the cornea (Krachmer, 1974; Cavanagh et al., 1976).

TABLE IV-2. — *Epithelial erosion syndrome*

A. *Recurrent erosions*
  1. Hereditary
  2. Spontaneous
  3. Post-traumatic
  4. Corneal dystrophies
  5. Nocturnal lagophthalmos

B. *Persistent aseptic epithelial defect*
  a. Post infective: metaherpetic, bacterial and fungal corneal ulcers.
  b. Post surgical: keratoplasty, cataract extraction.
  c. Neuroparalytic:
      Trigeminal denervation
      Facial paralysis
  d. Corneal burns:
      Chemical burns
      Thermokeratoplasty
  e. Bullous keratopathy
  f. Dry eyes
  g. Degenerations of cornea:
      — Salzman's nodular degeneration
      — Terrein's marginal degeneration
      — band keratopathy

Kaufman (1964) suggested that the pathogenesis of recurrent erosions and erosions of metaherpetic keratitis may be similar, as in both instances the basic defect lies in the basement membrane. Although we agree that the basic problem in both conditions is the lack of attachment of the epithelium due to a basement membrane defect, yet the pathogenesis may be different. Clinically, the corneal sensitivity is generally normal in recurrent erosions and reduced or absent in aseptic defects. Cellular alterations are common in aseptic defects. These alterations may result from corneal denervation, thermal and chemical burns (Duke-Elder and Leigh, 1965; Dohlman, 1978) or induced by herpes simplex virus (Maudgal and Misotten, 1979). In their histopathological study, Cavanagh et al. (1976) demonstrated the loss of cell polarity of the epithelium cells in aseptic defects. On the contrary, there is no conclusive evidence that such alterations of epithelium exist in recurrent erosions before the lesion develops, even though the dystrophic nature of the epithelium may be suspected. Finally, in aseptic defects we know that the destruction of basement membrane is not the primary change, but occurs after the destruction of epithelial cells due to various causes, while in recurrent erosions it is likely that the basement membrane changes antedate the epithelial edema.

Goldberg et al. (1974) have emphasized the role of cyclic AMP and cyclic GMP in their " Yin-Yang " hypothesis of biological regulation. It was proposed that the effect of cholinergic stimulation via cyclic GMP, is opposite to the effect of cyclic AMP or substances like catecholamines and prostaglandines leading to intracellular cyclic AMP accumulation. On the basis of this hypothesis and the experimental work (Johnson et al., 1972; Cavanagh, 1975), it is suggested that the increased intracellular cyclic AMP levels inhibit mitotic activity, cell locomotion and perhaps cause an increase in the basal lamina production. The cell glycogen levels are decreased. On the other hand, increased cyclic GMP has the opposite effect. Cavanagh et al. (1976), therefore, proposed that the humoral factors like catecholamines and prostaglandines associated with inflammatory process would discourage cell regeneration and cholinergic agents would encourage it. They also supposed that the worst inhibition of epithelial healing would occur when the inflammatory factors which increase cellular cyclic AMP levels are simultaneously present with decreased cholinergic levels in neurotrophic eyes. In their experience, this combination was present to some degree in all cases of persistent epithelial defects, and most pronounced in herpetic, chemical burn and dry eye cases, which combined neurotrophic effects with intense inflammation.

Treatment

Current treatment of the aseptic epithelium defects is similar to that of recurrent erosions. In addition, topical corticosteroids and anticollagenases may be helpful in metaherpetic and corneal burn cases, but should be used judiciously due to the increased risk of stromal melting and perforation with their use (Kaufman, 1964; Krachmer, 1974). Soft or scleral lenses are of value in large erosions.

However, when an aseptic epithelial defect remains stable for days and weeks, and the epithelium seems unable to close the erosion despite the above mentioned treatment; this inhibition of growth may be due either to the presence of substances that paralyze cell proliferation or prevent cell adhesion, or to the absence of agents necessary for normal epithelial proliferation as proposed by Cavanagh et al. (1976). If this hypothesis of the control mechanism of epithelial growth and proliferation is correct, two therapeutic approaches are justified in the treatment of persistent epithelial defects.

A hypothetic excess of inhibitory agents should be treated by irrigation. We prescribe irrigation with Hartmann® solution, copiously floading the eye every hour with 50 to 100 ml fluid through an infusion set. The use of continuous irrigation, by an irrigating contact lens, was less successful in our hands. This treatment, in the absence of any other medication, was very helpful in a number of patients; especially in torpid metaherpetic central epithelial defects in eyes with long standing disease, usually complicated with allergic reactions to one or more collyria. It was ineffective in some other cases, most markedly in deep marginal ulcers with a swollen conjunctival wall and active inflammation as seen in Mooren's ulcer and similar diseases.

A healing defect due to a hypothetic shortage of some substance should be treated with blepharorrhaphy. Embedding the erosion in a body cavity, surrounded on all sides with healthy epithelium, should compensate any local absence of essential substances. This, however, applies only to persistent erosions of unknown etiology.

The epithelial erosion due to exposure should be covered with conjunctival flap or soft contact lens, and those due to invasion of micro organismes should be treated with adequate antibiotics. The erosions accompanied by chronic inflammatory cell infiltration should be treated with adequate doses of corticosteroids.

For all other persistent epithelial defect we recommend irrigation therapy during 4 days to one week. If this therapy does not succeed, temporary blepharorrhaphy should be done.

BIBLIOGRAPHY

Bron, A.J. and Tripathi, R.C. — Cystic disorders of the corneal epithelium. I. Clinical aspects. *Brit. J. Ophthal.*, *57*, 361, 1973.
Cavanagh, H.D. — Herpetic ocular disease: Therapy of persistent epithelial defects. *Int. Ophthal. Clin.*, *15*, 67, 1975.
Cavanagh, H.D., Philaja, D., Thoft, A. and Dohlman, C.H. — The pathogenesis and treatment of persistent epithelial defects. *Trans. Amer. Acad. Ophthal. Otolaryngol.*, *81*, 754, 1976.
Dohlman, C.H. — The epithelial changes. Round table discussion on corneal diseases. *XXIII International Congress of Ophthalmology*, Kyoto 1978.
Duke-Elder, S. and Leigh, A.G. — System of Ophthalmology. Vol. VIII. Diseases of the outer eye. Part 2. Duke-Elder, S. (Ed.). Henry Kimpton, 1965.
Flynn, M.A. and Esterly, D.B. — Bilateral recurrent erosion of cornea. *Amer. J. Ophthal.*, *62*, 964, 1966.
Franceschetti, A. — Hereditäre rezidivierende Erosion der Hornhaut. *Z. Augenheilk.*, *66*, 309, 1928.
Franceschetti, A. and Klein, D. — In: *Genetics and Ophthalmology* Ed. Waardenburg. P.J. Franceschetti, A. and Klein, D.E. Vol. I, von Gorcum, Assen, 462, 1961.
Franke — Über Erkrankungen des Epithels der Hornhaut. *Klin. Mbl. Augenheilk.*, *44*, 508, 1906.
Gifford, S.R. — Epithelial dystrophy and recurrent erosion of the cornea as seen with the slit lamp. *Arch. Ophthal.*, *54*, 217, 1925.
Goldberg, N.D., Haddox, M.K., Dunham, E. et al. — The Yin-Yang hypothesis of biological control: opposing influences of cyclic GMP and cyclic AMP in the regulation of cell proliferation and other biological processes. Clarkson, B., Baserga, R., Eds. Cold Spring Harbor Press, 1974.
Goldman, J.N., Dohlman, C.H. and Kravitt, B.A. — The basement membrane of the human cornea in recurrent epithelial erosion syndrome. *Trans. Amer. Acad. Ophthal. Otolaryngol.*, *73*, 471, 1969.
Hansen — *Hospital Tidende*, *15*, 201, 1872.
Hermann, C. — La dystrophie grillagée de la cornée. *Ophthal.*, *112*, 350, 1946.
Hirstch, C. — Über die Sogen. recidivierende Erosion der Hornhaut (Arlt) und ihre Behandlung. *Wschr. Ther. Hyg. Anges*, *1*, 161, 1898.
Johnson, G.S., Morgan, W.D. and Pastan, I. — Regulation of cell motility by cyclic AMP. *Nature*, *235*, 54, 1972.
Kaufman, H.E. — Epithelial erosion syndrome: Metaherpetic keratitis. *Amer. J. Ophthal.*, *57*, 983, 1964.
Kenyon, K.R. — The synthesis of basement membrane by the corneal epithelium in bullous keratopathy. *Invest. Ophthal.*, *8*, 156, 1969.
Khodadoust, A.A. — Technique for the preparation of sheets of pure corneal epithelium. *Amer. J. Ophthal.*, *63*, 842, 1967.
Khodadoust, A.A., Silverstein, A.M., Kenyon, K.R. and Dowling, J.E. — Adhesion of regenerating corneal epithelium. *Amer. J. Ophthal.*, *65*, 339, 1968.
Krachmer, J.H. — Aseptic corneal erosions and ulcerations. In: *Current concepts in Ophthalmology*, Vol. IV. Ed. Blodi, F.C. The C.V. Mosby Company, 1974.
Maudgal, P.C. and Missotten, L. — Histopathology of the superficial herpes simplex keratitis. *Brit. J. Ophthal.*, *62*, 46, 1978.
Maudgal, P.C. and Missotten, L. — Histopathology and histochemistry of the superficial corneal epithelium in experimental herpes simplex keratitis. *Alb. v. Graefes Arch. Klin. exp. Ophthal.*, *209*, 239, 1979.
Maudgal, P.C. and Missotten, L. — Clinical and histological study of recurrent corneal erosions (in preparation).

Polack, F.M. — Contributions of electron microscopy to the study of corneal pathology. *Survey of Ophthal.*, *20*, 376, 1976.

Procksch, M. — Beitrag zur Klinik und Therapie der rezidivierenden Hornhauterosion. *Klin. Mbl. Augenheilk.*, *77*, 383, 1926.

Rodrigues, M.M. and Laibson, P.R. — Recurrent corneal erosions. *Trans. Pennsyl. Ac. Ophthal. Otolaryngol.*, *171*, 1976.

Salus, R. — Über traumatische und nichttraumatische rezidivierende Epithelerkrankung der Hornhaut. *Klin. Mbl. Augenheilk.*, *68*, 673, 1922.

Spektor, S. — Klinisches zur Frage der Ätiologie von doppelseitigen rezidivierende Erosionen der Hornhaut. *Klin. Mbl. Augenheilk.*, *87*, 661, 1931.

Sturrock, G.D. — Nocturnal lagophthalmos and recurrent erosion. *Brit. J. Ophthal.*, *60*, 97, 1976.

von Szily sen. — Über Disjunktion des Hornhautepithels. *von Graefes Arch. f. Ophthal.*, *51*, 486, 1900.

Triphati, R.C. and Bron, A.J. — Ultrastructural study of non-traumatic recurrent corneal erosion. *Brit. J. Ophthal.*, *56*, 73, 1972.

Tripathi, R.C. and Bron, A.J. — Cystic disorders of the corneal epithelium. II. Pathogenesis. *Brit. J. Ophthal.*, *57*, 376, 1973.

Trobe, J.D. and Laibson, P.R. — Dystrophic changes in the anterior cornea. *Arch. Ophthal.*, *87*, 378, 1972.

Valle, O. — Hereditary recurring corneal erosions. A familial study with special reference to Fuchs dystrophy. *Acta Ophthal.*, *45*, 829, 1967.

Wales, H.J. — A family history of corneal erosions. *Trans. Ophthal. Soc. N.Z.*, *8*, 77, 1955.

CHAPTER V

FILAMENTARY KERATITIS

Filamentary keratitis or keratopathy is a common condition characterised by the development of thin epithelial mucoid tags, sometimes upto one centimeter in length, attached to the corneal or perilimbal conjunctival surface from their upper end and a freely floating lower end.

Etiology

Filament formation occurs in many edematous, inflammatory and degenerative states of the cornea and may become chronic or recurrent (Duke-Elder and Leigh, 1965). Viral infections, particularly those manifesting as superficial punctate keratitis due to adenovirus, herpes and vaccinia, are typically associated with filamentary keratitis. Development of filaments in bacterial infections has not been described.

Epithelial filaments may develop after corneal trauma and edema due to various causes. Recurrent erosions (Wright, 1975; Maudgal et al., 1979) and erosions due to contact lens wear (Dada and Zisman, 1975) may precede filament formation.

Eye patching after surgery involves edematous and traumatic factors. Filaments may form after cataract operation, irrespective of the surgical technique, suture material or the use of chymotrypsin (Menezo et al., 1975; Dodds and Laibson, 1972). Epithelial edema may result from hypotonicity of tears due to lack of evaporation in prolonged patching of the eye (Cotlier, 1975). Filamentary keratitis associated with chronic blepharospasm (Wright, 1975) may arise due to similar factors.

In degenerative conditions, dry eyes of any etiology (Duke-Elder and Leigh, 1965; Glässer and Pietruschka, 1971; Wright, 1975; Maudgal, 1976; Maudgal et al., 1979) and superior limbic keratoconjunctivitis (Wright, 1975) are typically associated with filament formation. Filaments may also appear in keratoconus, neuroparalytic keratitis, benign mucus membrane pemphigoid and psoriasis (Dodds and Laibson, 1972).

Toxic and allergic factors may play an etiological role in the use of certain ocular drugs (Chassaing, 1968; Rüger, 1970; Brückner, 1974); the papillary conjunctivitis (Liebman, 1955; Maudgal et al., 1979); and chalazion of the eyelid (Wright, 1975). Filamentary keratitis has also been described in Osler-Weber-Rendu disease (Wolper and Laibson, 1969); aniridia and ocular albinism (Wright, 1975). They may arise as a complication of chronic uveitis due to sarcoidosis (Duke-Elder and Leigh, 1965).

Clinical picture

The signs and symptoms of filamentary keratitis are marked discomfort, irritation and foreign body sensation, accompanied by redness of the eye, photophobia, blepharospasm and frequent blinking. Except in severely affected cases of keratoconjunctivitis sicca, there is increased lacrimation. In dry eyes, both eyes may be involved.

On *biomicroscopy*, the number, size and shape of the filaments vary widely (fig. V-1). They originate from a localized triangular elevated area of conjunctiva or cornea with a greyish epithelial opacity underneath. A gutter like depression in the epithelium may be present at

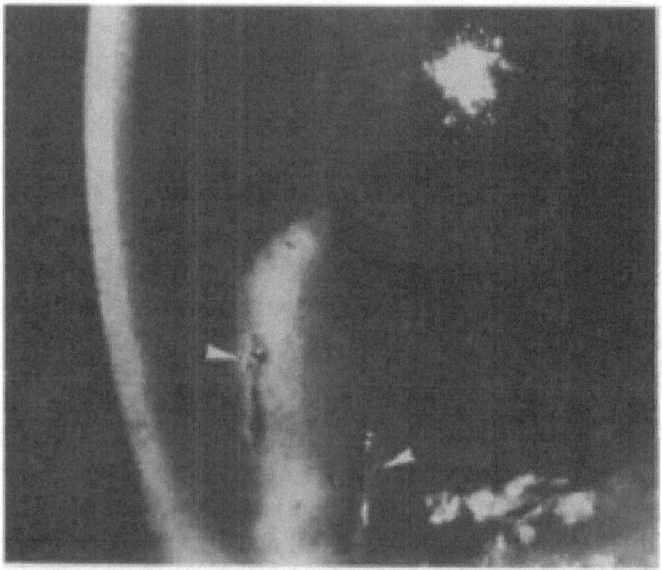

Fig. V-1. — Corneal filaments (arrows) in keratoconjunctivitis sicca.

their base. The freely floating lower end is somewhat thicker and globular. The filaments stain with fluorescein and rose bengal. They may fall off spontaneously but tend to recur. The corneal surface free of filaments may be apparently normal or show fine to coarse punctate epithelial opacities or semitransparent prominences.

Histopathology and pathogenesis

Histopathologically, filaments contain degenerated epithelium cells and mucoid material, which stain with alcian blue and PAS and give positive birefringence under polarisation microscopy (Wright, 1975; Maudgal et al., 1979). The bulb of the filament may contain variable amount of lipids, probably derived from meibomian secretions, but also, at least partly, from ointments as part of their medication (Wright, 1975).

Histologically (figs. V-2, V-3 and V-4), elongated superficial epithelium cells converge towards the stem of the filament at its base (Maudgal et al., 1979). These cells are edematous and show degenerative changes. The stem of the filament has a short torsional area, just after its origin, followed by an elongated bulbous expansion. Beyond this bulb, the stem becomes markedly thin with irregular thickenings containing degenerated cells. The terminal bulbs lack any cellular details. They are composed of degenerated cells and mucoid material. In keratoconjunctivitis sicca the filaments are shorter and thicker, lacking the torsional area and bulbous expansion.

The corneal surface devoid of filaments shows areas of focal degeneration with some mucoid material sticking to the cells. The epithelial cells surrounding the degeneration area slide towards the center of degeneration, as happens in the healing of epithelial pinprick injuries.

Reviewing the literature on filamentary keratitis, Duke-Elder and Leigh (1965), Thiel et al. (1972), and Wright (1975) have described three possible theories about the origin of filaments. The first and most accepted view is that of epithelial origin. The second hypothesis is the filament formation due to a defect in the subepithelial structures. Weskamp (1956) suggested that the superficial stromal layers were primarily involved in filamentary keratitis, while Thiel et al. (1972), on the basis of their electron microscopic study, proposed that the filaments develop from a basic defect in the attachment of the basement membrane to the Bowman's layer. According to the third

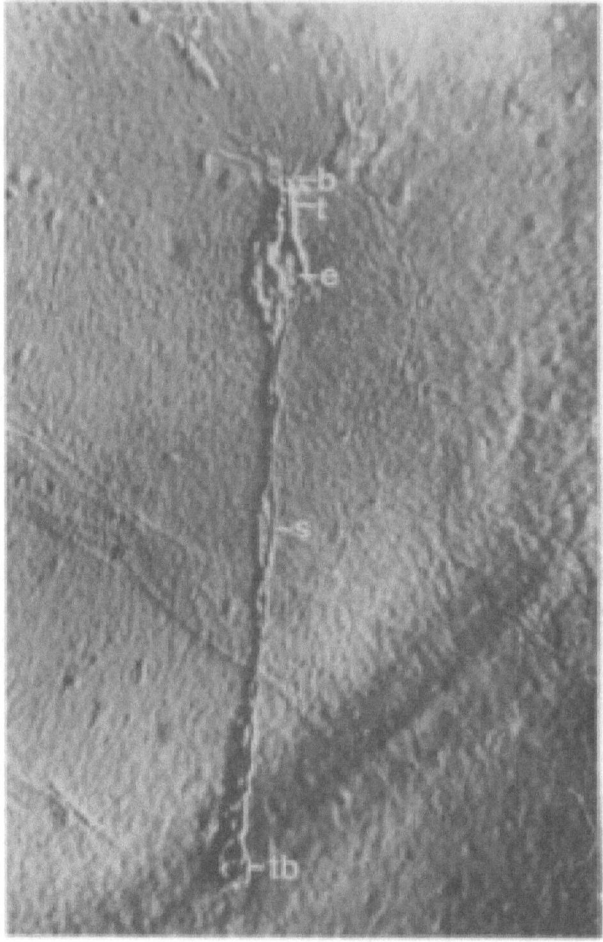

Fig. V-2. — Corneal filament in recurrent erosion; b: base, t: torsional area, e: bulbous expansion, s: stem, tb: terminal bulb. Oblique illumination microscopy of the replica. ×61.5. (From: Maudgal et al. Alb. v. Graefes Arch. Ophthal., 1979).

theory, currently favored by Wright (1975), filaments develop primarily from mucus and any epithelial involvement is secondary.

Our histopathological study by replica technique (Maudgal et al., 1979) indicates that the primary defect in filamentary keratitis is the focal degeneration of superficial epithelium. Some mucoid material apparently derived from conjunctival goblet cells sticks to the degenerated cells. The surrounding cells begin to slide towards the focus of degeneration to cover these small defects. The advancing edges of

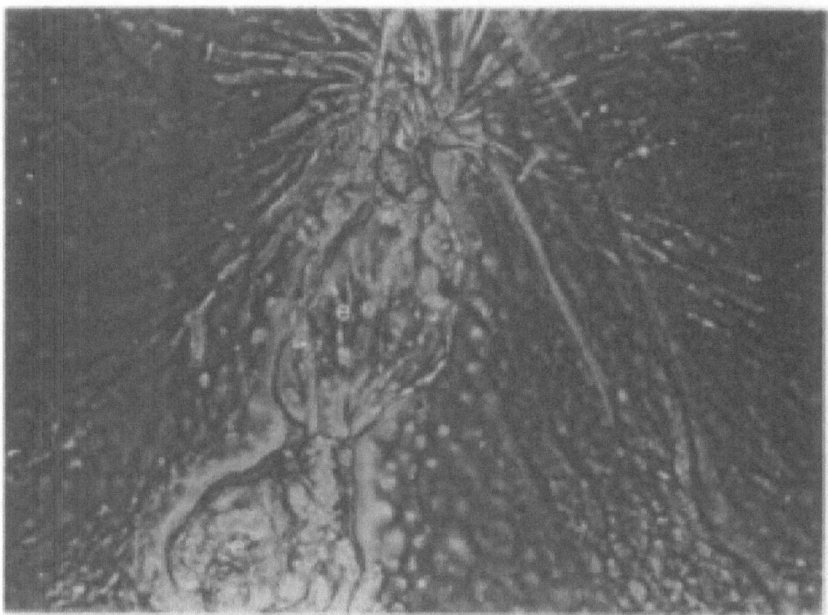

Fig. V-3. — Part of a filament showing elongated cells at the base (b), torsional area (t), and the expanded bulb (e). Phase contrast microscopy of the replica. × 130.

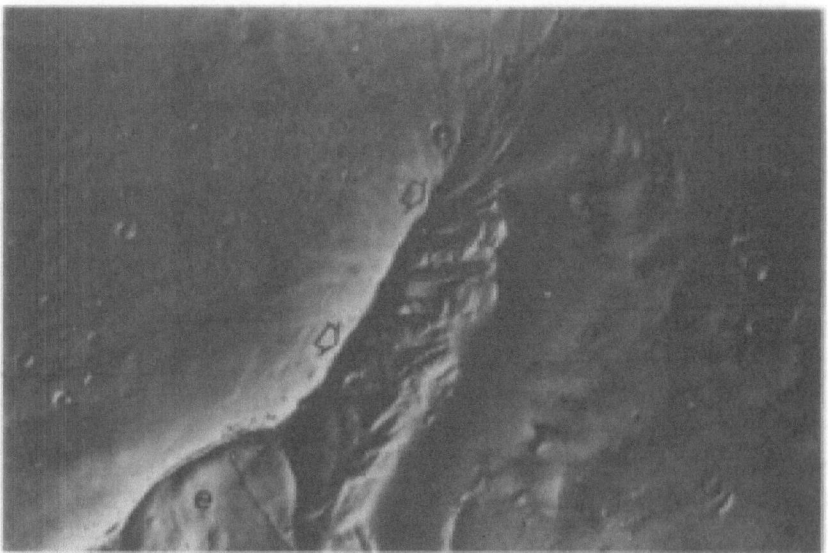

Fig. V-4. — Corneal filament at the limbus in a case of keratoplasty. The base (b) contains elongated cells followed by the torsional area (arrows) and bulbous expansion (e). Oblique illumination microscopy. × 130.

the converging cells are also covered with mucus, raising a small protuberance on the corneal surface. Somehow, the contact inhibition of the sliding cells does not take place, which stops the migration of the normal cells when the epithelium defect is closed. The presence of mucus or some other humoral factors may be responsible for the inhibition of this phenomenon. The continued sliding of the surrounding cells pushes the center of the protuberance upwards and the filament begins to grow from the corneal surface.

As the epithelial cells in the filament are displaced from their normal anatomical site, their physiological functions and metabolism suffer, resulting in their rapid degeneration. In dry eyes this degeneration is likely to occur much more quickly as the epithelial cells are already keratinised (Maudgal, 1976; Maudgal and Missotten, 1978). This mass of degenerated cells and mucus probably sticks to other degenerated cells which are abundant in keratoconjunctivitis sicca. Such attachments and also their shortness may be responsible for the absence of torsional area in the filaments of dry eyes.

The torsion of the filament is probably produced by the lid movements as proposed by other authors. The closure of palpebral aperture commences at the lateral canthus and ends at the medial canthus during a physiological blink (Anantanarayana, 1949). This uniform motion of the lids could be responsible for the direction of torsion. We found the same direction of torsion in all filaments in cases having multiple filaments.

The bulbous expansion following torsional area could be produced by the extension of the torsional portion of the filament into non torsional area. The irregular thickness of the stem probably depends on its extensibility and the traction put on it during lid movement.

The terminal bulb is the part which originated first from the epithelium and is likely to contain a greater amount of degenerated cells and mucoid material.

Wright (1975) has put forward the theory of "mucus receptor sites" for the development of filaments and contends that their origin is mainly from mucus. The mucus receptor sites, as described by Wright, have been shown as partly detached degenerating and piled up keratinised cells and keratin filaments in KCS (Maudgal 1976, Maudgal and Missotten, 1978). Mucus filaments extend between degenerated cells in the cases of KCS (Maudgal et al., 1979).

However, these filaments are very thin and do not represent the clinically recognised filamentary keratitis.

That the filaments originate from the subepithelial layers of the cornea is also unlikely as filamentary keratitis heals after making a replica. If there was a defect at the level of attachment of the basement membrane to Bowman's membrane or in superficial stroma, healing should not occur. In the study of Thiel et al. (1972) the filaments were mechanically pulled off for the microscopic study, which could have altered anatomical relations. The basal membrane like structures, described by them in the core of the filament, could have been the degenerated epithelial elements and mucus. The alteration in basal membrane itself could be the result of focal epithelial degeneration.

Treatment

Treatment of filamentary keratitis should be directed to the underlying etiological conditions, whenever it can be detected. Emolients and ointments should be avoided as they stick to the filaments increasing their size. Mechanical debridement of the epithelium may be sometimes helpful. A corneal replica (Missotten and Maudgal, 1977) may be used to remove the filaments after which the underlying disorder should be treated (Maudgal et al., 1979). Painting the area of filaments with 0,5% silver nitrate solution, after their mechanical removal, may ameliorate symptoms (Dodds and Laibson, 1972). Acetylcysteine, a mucolytic agent, in 20% aquous solution is recently being advocated (Wright, 1975).

In our experience 1% aquous solution of alum is frequently effective in the treatment of filamentary keratitis (unpublished data), but irritates the eye like acetylcystein.

BIBLIOGRAPHY

Anantanarayna, A. — Note on the mechanisme of eyelid closure in blinking. *Proc. All. India Ophthal. Soc.*, *10*, 154, 1949.
Brückner, R. — Über Fächenbildungen am Hornhautepithel. *Klin. Mbl. Augenheilk.*, *164*, 130-133, 1974.
Cotlier, E. — The Cornea. Adlers physiology of the eye. Ed. Moses, R.A., The C.V. Mosby Company, St. Louis 1975.
Chassaing, M.J. — La kératite filamenteuse est-elle une manifestation allergique particulière à l'épithélium cornéen? *Bull. Soc. Ophtal. Fr.*, *68*, 912, 1968.
Dada, V.K. and Zisman, F. — Contact lens induced filamentary keratitis. *Amer. J. Optom. Physiol. Optics*, *52*, 545, 1975.

Dodds, H.T. and Laibson, P.R. — Filamentary keratitis following cataract extraction. *Arch. Ophthal.*, *88*, 609, 1972.

Duke-Elder, S. and Leigh, A.G. — System of Ophthalmology, Vol. VIII, Diseases of the outer eye. Ed. Duke-Elder, S., Henry Kimpton, London, 1965.

Gläser, W. and Pietruschka, G. — Beitrag zur Symptomatik und zum klinischen Verlauf der Keratitis filiformis unter besonderer Berücksichtigung des Sjögren-Syndrome. *Zschr. Ärztl. Fortbild.*, *65*, 720, 1971.

Leber, T. — Präparate zu dem Vortrag über Entstehung der Netzhautablösung und über verschiedene Hornhautaffecktionen. *Ber. Ophthal. Ges. Heidelberg*, *14*, 165, 1882.

Liebman, S.D. — An unusual case of filamentary keratitis. *Arch. Ophthal.*, *54*,. 434, 1955.

Maudgal, P.C. — The epithelial response in keratitis sicca and keratitis herpetica (an experimental and clinical study). Doctoral thesis University of Leuven, 1976. Documenta Ophthalmologica, 45: 223, 1978.

Maudgal, P.C. and Missotten, L. — Cytology of the superficial keratinised cells in experimenal keratitis sicca. *Ophthalmologica*, *176*, 113, 1978.

Maudgal, P.C., Missotten, L. and Van Deuren, H. — Study of filamentary keratitis by replica technique. *Alb. v. Graefes Arch. exp. Klin. Ophthal.*, *211*, 11, 1979.

Menezo, J.L., Suares, R. und Menezo, V. — Verbleibende Irislähmung und keratitis filiformis: Seltene Komplikationen nach kataraktoperationen. *Klin. Mbl. Augenheilk.*, *166*, 523, 1975.

Missotten, L. and Maudgal, P.C. — The corneal replica technique used to study the superficial corneal epithelium in vivo. *Amer. J. Ophthal.*, *84*, 104, 1977.

Rüger, K. — Keratitis filiformis nach links-glaucosan. *Klin. Monatsbl. Augenheilk.*, *157*, 825, 1970.

Thiel, H.J., Blümcke, S. und Kessler, W.D. — Zur pathogenese der Keratopathia filamentose (Keratitis filiformis) Licht und elektronenmikroskopische Untersuchung. *Alb. von Graefes Arch. Klin. exp. Ophthal.*, *184*, 330, 1972.

Weskamp, C. — Parenchrymatous origin of filamentary keratitis. *Amer. J. Ophthal.*, *42*, 115, 1956.

Wolper, J. and Laibson, P.R. — Hereditary hemorrhagic telangiectasis (Rendu-Osler-Weber disease) with filamentary keratitis. *Arch. Ophthal.*, *81*, 272, 1969.

Wright, P. — Filamentary keratitis. *Trans. Ophthal. Soc. U.K.*, *95*, 260, 1975.

CHAPTER VI

FINE PUNCTATE EPITHELIAL KERATITIS

In the classification of punctate keratitis, Duke-Elder (1965) characterised the fine punctate keratitis as the superficial punctate white or opaque lesions visible without any stain on the cornea. However, the involved cells stain irregularly with fluorescein and rose bengal.

Fine punctate keratitis is seen in many conditions of diverse etiology (table VI-1). In this chapter we shall discuss warts and molluscum contagiosum infections which are two important causes of chronic unilateral keratoconjunctivitis. Other major conditions are discussed under appropriate headings in this report.

TABLE VI-1. — *Conditions associated with fine punctate keratitis*

a) Bacterial: Staphylococcal blepharoconjunctivitis
b) Viral: Herpes simplex
       Herpes zoster
       Molluscum contagiosum
       Warts
c) Chlamydial: Trachoma
           Inclusion conjunctivitis
d) Allergic: Vernal keratoconjunctivitis
       Drug allergy
e) Photoactinic and irradiational keratoconjunctivitis
f) Dry eyes: Keratoconjunctivitis sicca
        Exposure keratitis
        Keratitis lagophthalmos
g) Iatrogenic: Toxic effects of ocular collyria
h) Unknown etiology: Rosacea
              Superior limbic keratoconjunctivitis

WARTS

Warts (verruca) are common horny growths on skin and sometimes on mucus membranes caused by a member of the papovavirus group. This DNA virus has a cubic symmetry and measures 40 to 55 nm in size. The virus is ether resistant and does not possess an envelope (Locatcher-Khorazo and Seegal, 1972; Pumper and Yama-shiroya, 1975). The virus has not been propagated in the laboratory. Like other members of the group it is oncogenic.

Epidemiology

Warts spread by direct contact from person to person or by indirect contact with contaminated objects. Autoinoculation helps the spread of the warts from one body site to another. Man is the only reservoir of this worldwide disease. Children and immunò-suppressed adults are commonly affected.

Pathogenesis and Pathology

The virus enters the skin and remains localized in it. Viremia does not occur.

Histological examination of the common wart (verruca vulgaris) shows hyperkeratosis with acanthosis, papillomatosis and parakerato-sis. The granular layer becomes hypertrophied. Large vacuolated cells are present in the outer layers of the stratum spinosum and granular layer. Cell vacuolation is much more in flat warts (verruca plana) while papillomatosis and parakeratosis are rare (Pumper and Yama-shiroya, 1975). Electron microscopy demonstrates abundant virus particles in the affected cells (Strauss et al., 1950; Melnick et al., 1952).

Clinical picture

Clinically warts are differentiated into many forms depending on the site of body involvement and the shape and appearance of the lesion. We are concerned here with common warts which may appear on any area of the body. They are raised and irregular cauli-flowerlike epidermal tumors occurring singly or in groups. Warts may be one millimeter to several millimeters in size.

Keratoconjunctivitis

Soft pink multiple papillomata having raspberry appearance may develop in the lower fornix at the inner canthus (Duke-Elder, 1965). Fedukowicz (1978) observed a cornu cutaneum about 3 cm in size, at the medial canthus.

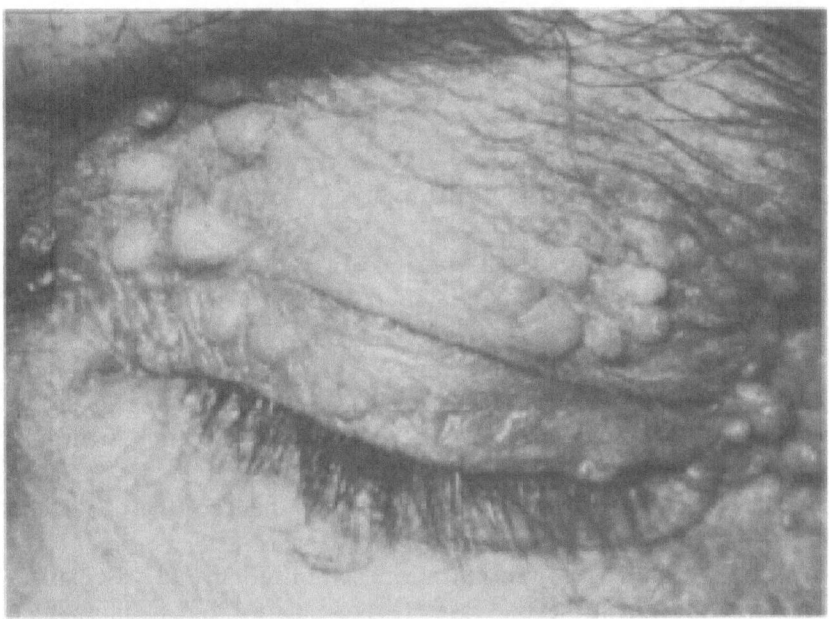

Fig. VI-1. — Multiple warts on the lids and lid margins.

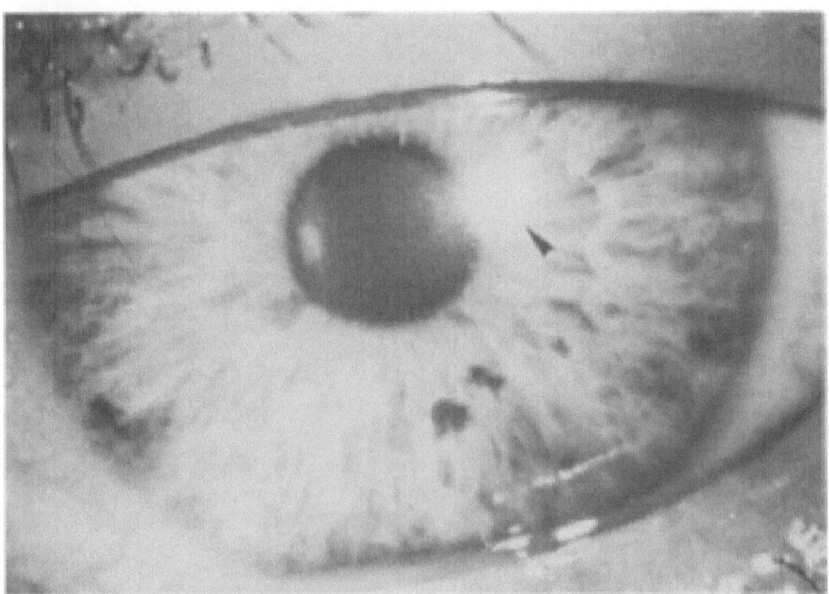

Fig. VI-2. — Warts keratoconjunctivitis. Ground glass appearance of the corneal surface is better visible in the pupillary area. Rough corneal surface scatters light (arrow).

Frequently, however, conjunctivitis or keratoconjunctivitis develops if the warts are situated at or near the lid margin (fig. VI-1) (de Roeth, 1939). They may be hidden between the cilia and are difficult to find unless a careful search is made.

Conjunctivitis is of subacute catarrhal type with scanty discharge. Generally, there is papillary hypertrophy of the conjunctiva but follicles may also develop.

Multiple punctate epithelial erosions may develop on the cornea accompanied by pain and photophobia (Duke-Elder, 1965; Fedukowicz, 1978).

We had the opportunity to see a case of bilateral verrucose keratitis with multiple verrucae of the eyelids and lid margins. One eye was more severely involved than the other. In addition to diffuse punctate epithelial erosions, we observed diffuse fine grey opaque punctate lesions of the superficial corneal epithelium (figs. VI-2 and VI-3) staining with fluorescein and rose bengal.

Corneal ulceration is rare but stromal infiltration and vascularisation may develop in severe cases (Duke-Elder, 1965). Conjunctival scrapings show only mononuclear cells. We have done preliminary

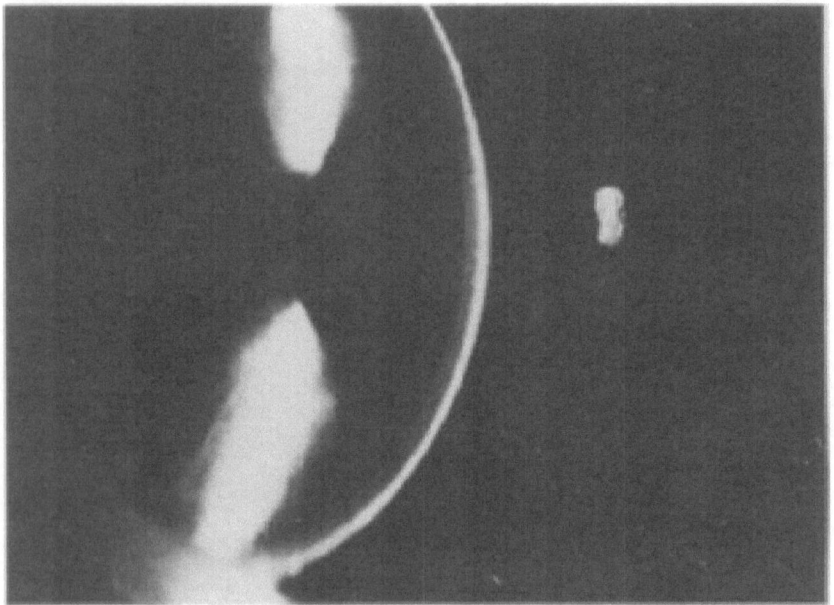

Fig. VI-3. — Slit beam picture of the eye in figure VI-2. The punctate opacification is limited to the epithelium.

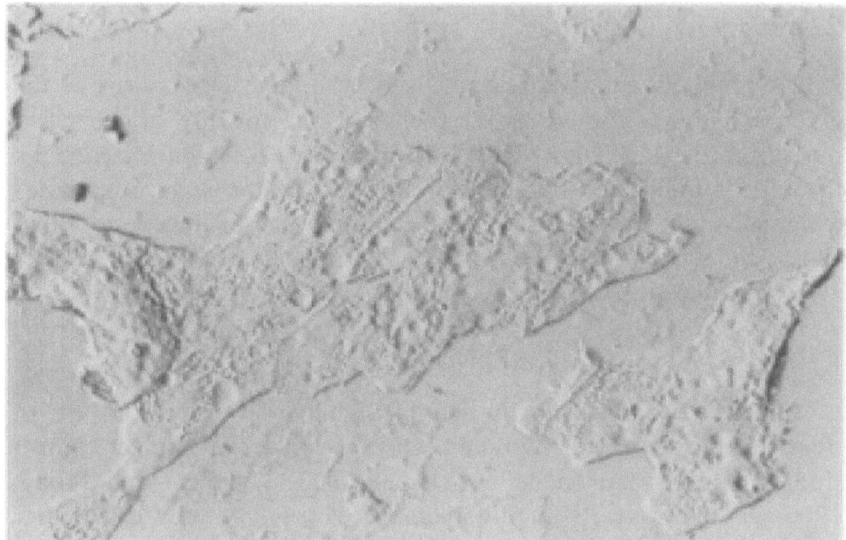

Fig. VI-4. — Superficial epithelial cells of the cornea show numerous bubble-like elevations on the surface in warts keratitis. Oblique illumination microscopy. × 520.

examination of the corneal replica of our patient. The corneal epithelial cells were irregularly arranged and varied in size. The nuclei were fragmented in many cells. The surfaces of numerous cells showed multiple bubble-like elevations (fig. VI-4). The size of the bubbles varied in the same cell. Some cells were more severely affected than others. We are not aware yet if virus is present in these cells. Further studies are in progress to clarify this point.

Most authors agree that keratoconjunctivitis is probably a toxic reaction to the warts on the lid margins.

Treatment

The only treatment of the verrucose keratoconjunctivitis is the removal of warts on the lids, which may be accomplished by surgical excision, electrocautery, cryocautery or chemical cautery. In our case, making the corneal replica did not affect the keratitis. It has been stated that warts may disappear on psychotherapy or suggestion (Allington, 1952). Spontaneous regression may also occur (Korting, 1973).

MOLLUSCUM CONTAGIOSUM

It is primarily a skin disease caused by a large DNA virus of the Poxvirus group. The virus is ether resisant, roughly brick-shaped measuring 230×300 nm (fig. VI-5). The disease is characterized by the raised umblicated nodules on any part of the skin. Sometimes conjunctiva and rarely cornea is the primary site of infection (Duke-Elder, 1965; Friedman-Kien, 1970; Locatcher-Khorazo and Seegal, 1972; Fedukowicz, 1978).

Epidemiology

Molluscum contagiosum is mainly a childhood disease limited to man. The virus spreads by direct physical contact or indirect contact through fomites (Julianelle and Janus, 1943; Overfield and Brody, 1966; Fedukowicz, 1978). Involvement of genitalia may occur after

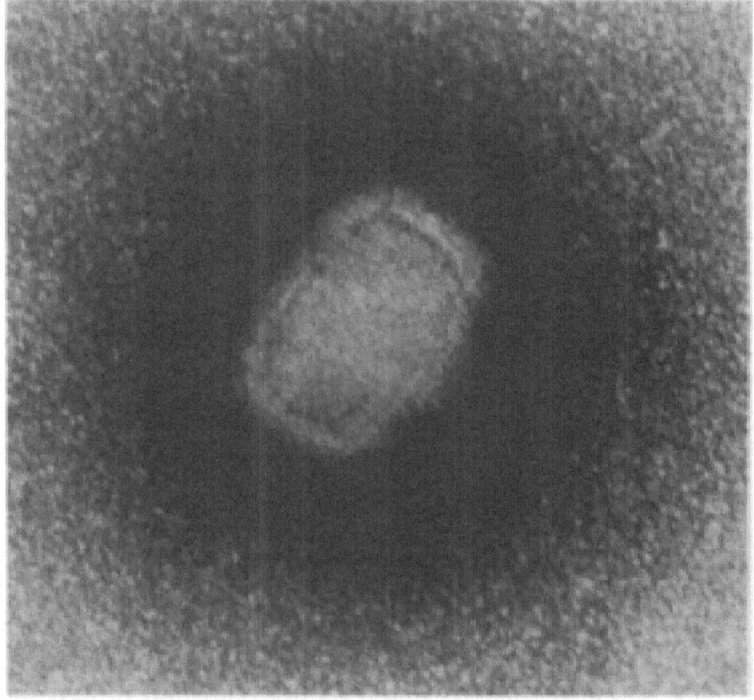

Fig. VI-5. — Electron microphotograph of the molluscum contagiosum virus under high magnification. Phosphotungstic acid negative staining. (Courtesy of Professor J. Desmeyter and Dr. G. De Groote).

sexual intercourse (Lynch and Minkin, 1968; Cobbold and Mac Donald, 1970). Attempts to culture the virus have been unsuccessful, but on inoculation of lesion extracts to human volunteers the disease appears in 2 weeks to 2 months (Friedman-Kien, 1970). Autoinoculation is frequent and leads to spread of the lesions.

Pathology

Histologically, the epithelial nodules are enveloped in a fibrous capsule, divided by septa containing aggregates of epithelial cells. Many of these cells become enormously enlarged. The nucleus is marginated and eventually destroyed. The cytoplasm is replaced by a large eosinophillic inclusion body (Duke-Elder, 1965; Fedukowicz, 1978; Grayson, 1979). Plenty of virus particles are present in the inclusion body as demonstrated by electron microscopy (Banfield et al., 1951).

Clinical picture

The molluscum contagiosum lesions appear as discrete raised, round pearly white papules; typically umblicated in the center and often showing a small dark spot. On squeezing cheesy material can easily be expressed from the papules. Atypical lesions in the form of sebaceous cyst, verruca or milium may, however, develop (Curtin and Theodore, 1955). The lesions vary in number and size i.e. from 1 mm to giant lesions measuring 2 cm in diameter (Meer Maastricht and Gomperts, 1950). Average size is about 4 mm. The papules persist generally from 6 months to 1 year, but may persist for several years. Trauma and secondary infection may cause resolution of the lesions. Spontaneous healing may take place without scarring (Friedman-Kien, 1970).

The skin of the face, especially the eyelids, is commonly involved. Other frequently affected sites are anogenital region and trunk.

Keratoconjunctivitis

Sometimes molluscum lesions may occur on the conjunctiva, especially the palpebral conjunctiva of the lower lid. Cornea is only exceptionally involved (Duke-Elder, 1965; Vannas and Lapinleima, 1967).

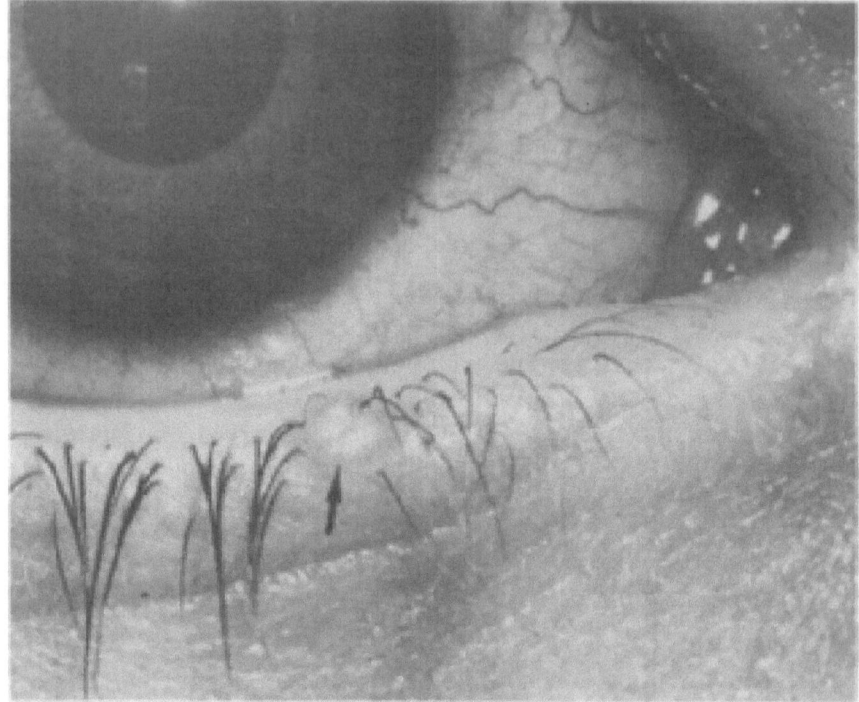

Fig. VI-6. — Molluscum contagiosum lesion at the lid margin (arrow).

Molluscum lesions of lid margins (fig. VI-6) give rise to an acute catarrhal conjunctivitis, which typically becomes chronic with follicle formation in the upper and lower fornices. In untreated cases corneal complications may develop. Punctate epithelial erosions, punctate epithelial and subepithelial keratitis involving the upper part of the cornea and pannus formation may develop (Lee, 1944; Magnus, 1944, Mathur, 1960; Balakrishnan, 1964; Vannas and Lapinleima, 1967).

Since the virus is not present in the conjunctival and corneal epithelium, keratoconjunctivitis is thought to be of toxic origin secondary to the lid infection.

Treatment

Treatment of the lid lesions by chemical cautery, electrocautery, cryotherapy, surgical excision or fulgration produces prompt relief of the skin as well as the eye condition.

BIBLIOGRAPHY

Allington, H.V. — Review of the psychotherapy of warts. *Arch. Dermatol.*, *66*, 316, 1952.

Balakrishnan, E. — Molluscum contagiosum conjunctivitis. *J. All. India Ophthal. Soc.*, *12*, 173, 1964.

Banfield, W.G., Bunting, H., Strauss, M.J., Melnick, J.L. — Electronmicrographs of thin sections of molluscum contagiosum. *Proc. Soc. Exp. Biol. Med.*, 77, 843, 1951.

Cobbold, R.J.D. and MacDonald, A. — Molluscum contagiosum as a sexually transmitted disease. *Practitioner*, *204*, 416, 1970.

Curtin, B.J. and Theodore, F.H. — Ocular molluscum contagiosum. *Amer. J. Ophthal.*, *39*, 302, 1955.

de Roetth, A.F. — Common wart as an etiological factor in certain cases of conjunctivitis and keratitis. *Arch. Ophthal.*, *21*, 409, 1939.

Duke-Elder, S. — System of ophthalmology, Vol. VIII, Diseases of the outer eye. Part 1, Henry Kimpton, London, 1965.

Fedukowicz, H.B. — External infections of the eye. Appleton-Century-Crofts. New York, 1978.

Friedman-Kien, A.E. — Minor viral diseases of the skin and mucosal surfaces. In: *Harrisons Principles of Internal Medicine*. McGraw-Hill Book Company, New York, 1970.

Grayson, M. — Disease of the cornea. The C.V. Mosby Company, London, 1979.

Julianelle, L.A. and Janus, W.M. — Molluscum contagiosum of the eye, its clinical course and transmissibility, and the cultivability of the virus. *Amer. J. Ophthal.*, *26*, 565, 1943.

Korting, G.W. — The skin and eye. W.B. Saunders Company, London, 1973.

Lee, O.S. Jr. — Keratitis occuring with molluscum contagiosum. *Arch. Ophthal.*, *31*, 64, 1944.

Locatcher-Khorazo, D. and Seegal, B.C. — Microbiology of the eye. The C.V. Mosby Company, St. Louis, 1972.

Lynch, P.J. and Minkin, W. — Molluscum contagiosum of the adult: probable venereal transmission. *Arch. Dermatol.*, *98*, 141, 1968.

Magnus, J.A. — Unilateral follicular conjunctivitis due to molluscum contagiosum. *Brit. J. Ophthal.*, *28*, 245, 1944.

Melnick, J.L., Bunting, H., Banfield, W.G., Strauss, M.J. and Gaylord, W.H. — Electron microscopy of viruses of human papilloma, molluscum contagiosum, and vaccinia, including observations on the formation of virus within the cells. *Ann. N.Y. Acad. Sci.*, *54*, 1214, 1952.

Mathur, S.P. — Ocular complications in molluscum contagiosum. *Brit. J. Ophthal.*, *44*, 572, 1960.

Meer Maastricht, B.C.J. vd and Gomperts, C.E. — Molluscum contagiosum giganteum. *Amer. J. Ophthal.*, *33*, 965, 1950.

Overfield, T.M. and Brody, J.A. — An epidemiological study of molluscum contagiosum in Anchorage. *Alaska, J. Pediat, 69*, 640, 1966.

Pumper, R. Wm. and Yamashiroya, H.M. — Essentials of medical virology. W.B. Saunders Company, London, 1975.

Strauss, M.J., Bunting, H. and Melnick, J.L. — Viruslike particles and inclusion bodies in skin papillomas. *J. Invest. Dermatol.*, *15*, 433, 1950.

Vannas, S. and Lapinleima, K. — Molluscum contagiosum in the skin, caruncle and conjunctiva. *Acta Ophthal.*, *45*, 314, 1967.

CHAPTER VII

COARSE PUNCTATE KERATITIS

Coarse punctate keratitis is primarily an epithelial disease producing grey or yellowish spotty lesions on the cornea due to the involvement of groups of epithelial cells. The spotty lesions may assume macular, areolar or stellate forms, and stain with fluorescein and rose bengal (Duke-Elder and Leigh, 1965). They may be associated with fine diffuse punctate keratitis. In many conditions a subepithelial component develops as the epithelial disease heals. Coarse punctate keratitis occurs in a wide variety of ocular disease. The major causes are enumerated in table VII-I.

TABLE VII-I. — *Causes of coarse punctate keratitis*

a) Virus diseases: Adenovirus
       Herpes simplex
       Herpes zoster
       Vaccinia
b) Chlamydia diseases: Trachoma
       TRIC punctate keratitis
c) Unknown etiology: Thygeson's superficial punctate keratitis
d) Infrequent causes: Ocular pemphigoid
       Keratoconjunctivitis sicca
       Ocular rosacea
       Vernal keratoconjunctivitis

Herpes virus infections and keratoconjunctivitis sicca are discussed elsewhere in this book. Three conditions: Adenovirus, Chlamydia infections; and Thygeson's superficial punctate keratitis are dealt with in this chapter.

ADENOVIRAL KERATOCONJUNCTIVITIS

Adenoviruses constitute a group of non-enveloped viruses having a DNA core surrounded by a protein coat or capsid in an icosahedral symmetry. The capsid has 252 surface subunits or capsomeres and measures 70 to 80 nm (fig. VII-1). Adenoviruses are ether resistant.

Adenoviruses are common pathogens of man with a world-wide distribution and tendency to grow in various epithelia. Rowe et al. (1953) first isolated a member of adenovirus group from the adenoid tissues of children. More than 30 other types have been isolated till now from the adenoid tissues, tonsils; nasal and throat washings; corneal and conjunctival scrapings; eye and anal swabbings and stools (Locatcher-Khorazo and Seegal, 1972). The distinction between the various types is made by reacting the isolated virus with standardized sera containing known antibodies against different types. Although the adenoviruses have been isolated from asymptomatic individuals (Huebner and Rowe, 1957; Vorgosko et al., 1965), they are a common cause of upper respiratory infections in children and adults. The eye becomes frequently involved leading to follicular conjunctivitis. Two distinct conditions, pharyngoconjunctival fever

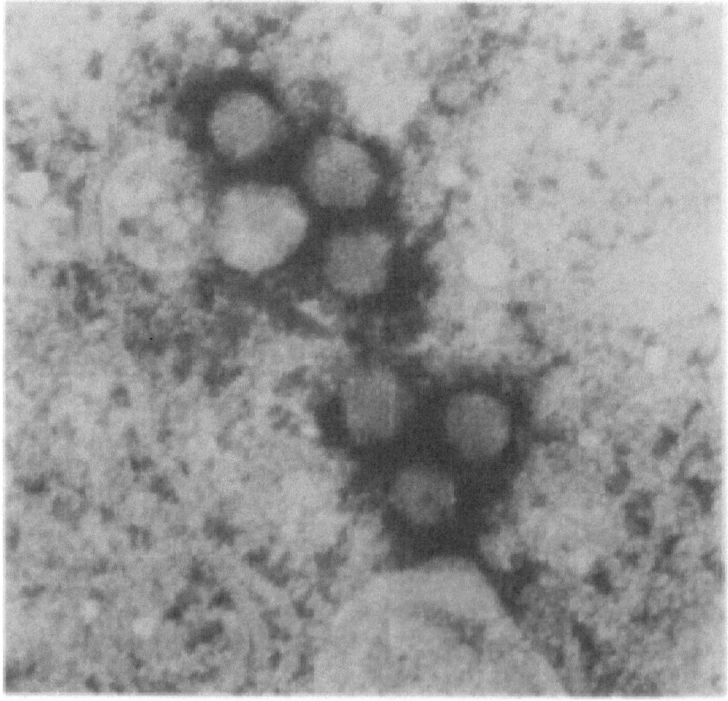

Fig. VII-1. — Adenoviruses seen under high magnification in a phosphotungstic acid stained preparation. Electron microscopy. (Courtesy of Prof. J. Desmeyter and Dr. G. De Groote).

and epidemic keratoconjunctivits, are important from ophthalmologist's point of view. Corneal involvement is characteristic in latter while transient superficial keratitis may develop in former.

PHARYNGOCONJUNCTIVAL FEVER

Pharyngoconjunctival fever was probably first described by Béal in 1907, but its association with adenoviruses was recognised only in the sixth decade of this century (Bell et al., 1955; and 1956; Bell 1957; Rowe et al., 1955; Fowle et al., 1955; Cockburn et al., 1956). Adenovirus type 3 is the most frequent invader, but other types (1, 4, 5, 6, 7, 7a, 9 and 14) may also produce mild to severe illness. (Bell et al., 1955; Ward et al., 1955; Fowle et al., 1955; Evans, 1957; Huebner and Rowe, 1957; Kendall et al., 1957; Kimura et al., 1957; Oker-Blom et al., 1957; Van der Veen and Van der Ploeg, 1958; Jones, 1962; Muzzi et al., 1975).

Epidemiology

Pharyngoconjunctival fever is a highly infectious, acute but transient disease, predominantly affecting children and young adults but may occur at any age. Sporadic cases (Kimura et al., 1957) and epidemic outbreaks have been described in families and schools. The epidemics spread through contact and swiming pools (Derrick, 1943; Cockburn et al., 1956; Ormsby and Aitchison, 1955; Okamura, 1960). Incubation period is 5 to 6 days.

Clinical picture

Duke-Elder (1965) characterizes this illness by a triad of symptoms: fever, pharyngitis and a non-purulent follicular conjunctivitis, often associated with regional lymphadenitis. The symptoms may appear singly or together in all grades of severity. Fever may be mild initially but rises rapidly to 39 °C or higher; accompanied by malaise, muscle pains, headache, abdominal discomfort and diarrhea. The posterior oropharynx is congested with follicle formation.

Ocular involvement

The most common feature of the pharyngoconjunctival fever is follicular conjunctivitis with preauricular adenopathy. The eyes become red with irritation and watering. Photophobia and blepharospasm are not pronounced. The eyelids become swollen. One eye is usually affected first but the infection may spread soon to the other eye. The discharge is usually serous and scanty but rarely mucopurulent.

On examination, the conjunctiva is markedly hyperaemic with chemosis. The follicle formation varies. Both the follicles and hyperemia are typically more marked on the lower lid and fornix than the upper (fig. VII-2). Conjunctival scrapings contain mononuclear inflammatory cells. Conjunctivitis may be initially associated with a superficial punctate keratitis which may become subepithelial before disappearing (Jones, 1962).

The illness may subside in 2 to 10 days (average 5 days) but sometimes complete healing may not occur untill after 3 weeks. The infecting virus, usually type 3, can be isolated from the conjunctival and pharyngeal swabbings or scrapings in the first few days of disease. Circulating specific antibodies have been detected for longer than 3 years after infection (Cockburn et al., 1956). Immunity is type specific. Recovery from infection with one type does not result in resistance to infection with other types (Locatcher-Khorazo and Seegal, 1972).

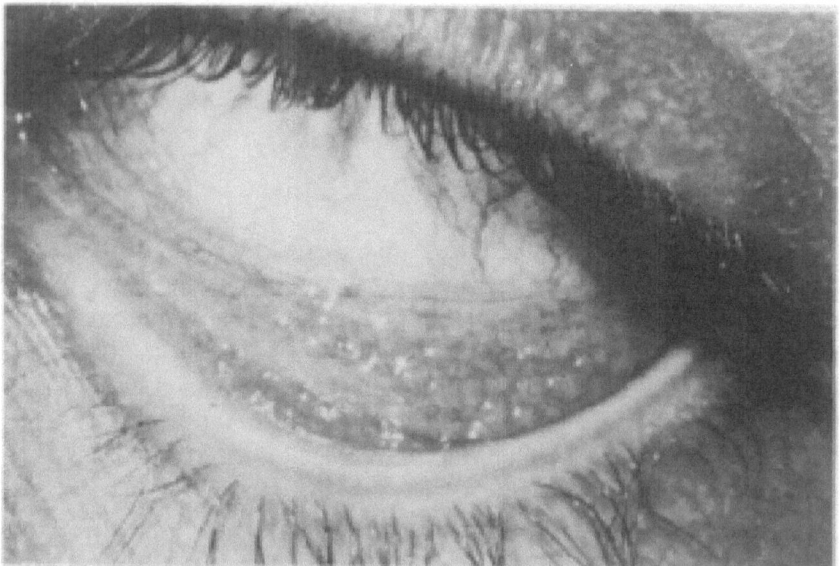

Fig. VII-2. — Large follicles on the inferior palpebral conjunctiva in adenovirus infection.

Treatment

Treatment of the condition is symptomatic. There is no specific therapy available.

EPIDEMIC KERATOCJUNCTIVITIS

Epidemic keratoconjunctivitis is characterized by the acute onset of a follicular conjunctivitis with regional lymphadenopathy, early superficial punctate keratitis followed by focal epithelial keratitis and delayed development of subepithelial corneal infiltrates during convalescence. Subconjunctival hemorrhages, conjunctival pseudomembranes and symblepharon may develop (Dawson et al., 1970; and 1972; Vastine et al., 1976).

Fuchs (1889) first described the clinical desease as "superficial punctate keratitis". In the same year Adler and von Reuss described the same illness, independently, as "keratitis subepithelialis" and "macular keratitis" (Duke-Elder, 1965). Subsequently, reports of epidemics and sporadic cases came from different parts of the world (Locatcher-Khorazo and Seegal, 1972). Hogan and Crawford (1942) suggested the readily adopted and still lingering term "epidemic keratoconjunctivitis" (EKC) to describe this disease.

Etiology

The etiological agent was first described as adenovirus type 8 (Jawetz et al., 1955).

Epidemic keratoconjunctivitis caused by type 8 adenovirus has been well studied by different authors (Bietti and Bruna, 1957; Jawetz et al., 1957; Leopold, 1957; Mitsui et al., 1957, 1959; Thygeson, 1957; Davidson, 1964; Imre et al., 1964; Marre et al., 1967; Laibson et al., 1968; Grist et al., 1970; Dawson et al., 1972; Hart et al., 1972; Freyler and Sehorst, 1975 and 1976; Chiba et al., 1976; Zweighaft et al., 1977 and many others). Other types of adenoviruses, i.e. 1 to 7, 9 to 16, 19 and 29 may cause moderate to severe keratoconjunctivitis clinically indistinguishable from that caused by type 8 virus (Bell, 1957; Hogan, 1957; Kimura et al., 1957; Ormsby et al., 1957; Sugiura et al., 1959; Jones, 1962, Tommila and Lapinleimu, 1965; Dawson et al., 1972; Germanis and Jeansson, 1973; Caldwell et al., 1974; Desmyter et al., 1974; Reid et al., 1974;

Hierholzer et al., 1974. Tanifuji et al., 1974; Guyer et al., 1975; Jackson et al., 1975; Wigand et al., 1975; Burns and Potter, 1976; O'Day et al., 1976; Vastine et al., 1976; Warring et al., 1976; Boni and Schmidt, 1977; Kàsova et al., 1977, Kàsova and Bruckova, 1977; Zografos, 1977; Tullo and Higgins, 1978 and others). Different types of adenoviruses have been isolated in mixed or simultaneous outbreaks (Reid et al., 1974; Wigand et al., 1975; Kàsova and Bruckova, 1977; and others).

Epidemiology

Large or limited outbreaks of EKC occur mostly in industrial plants; hospitals and crowded communities. Many outbreaks have been traced to ophthalmologist's office and eye care centers. Boni and Schmidt (1977) reported a small self-induced outbreak due to type 19 adenovirus in a correctional facility for young boys. Although epidemics are frequent, sporadic cases with clinically typical picture of epidemic-form may occur (Fowle et al., 1957; Hirota, 1957; Koseki, 1960; Profeta et al., 1963; Grayston et al., 1964; Jansco and Simons, 1965; Grist et al., 1970; Knopf and Hierholzer, 1975; and others). Sporadic cases are commonly caused by types 3, 7 and 19.

EKC is a highly contagious disease spreading by person to person contact. Contaminated hands of ophthalmologists and instruments, especially Schiotz tonometers, are known to transmit the virus to different patients. Sporadic cases may occur by finger to eye transmission from subclinical upper respiratory tract infections. Why some infections assume epidemic forms, and others remain limited to small outbreaks or occur sporadically, is not clear. However, the biological differences among different types of viruses are not ruled out. Golden et al. (1971) detected an inhibitory factor which suppressed the cytopathogenic effects and reduced the infectivity of the virus in vitro. A larger quantity of this factor was isolated from non epidemic strain than the epidemic strain.

The incubation period ranges from 2 to 14 days. Generally, acute symptoms appear 7 to 9 days after infection. adult population between 20 and 40 years is commonly affected but the disease has been described at 2 months and 85 years of age. Males are about twice more commonly affected than females. Except type 7 adenovirus infections, which are frequent in summer months, there is no seasonal variation. Systemic symptoms of mild pharyngitis and rhinitis may precede the onset of EKC.

Clinical picture

The *ocular involvement* is typically acute and involves one eye in about 70% cases. At the onset, only the *conjunctiva* seems to be involved. The eye becomes red with moderate to severe swollen eyelids, with a feeling of discomfort, irritation or foreign body sensation. Pain and variable photophobia may be associated. Because of the typical symptoms, the disease has been called the "pink eye" (or "shipyard eye" because of the epidemics in shipyard workers). The conjunctiva, caruncle and plica semilunaris are also edematous and red, but these symptoms are not typical for EKC. (Wigand et al., 1975). Petechial and sometimes diffuse subconjunctival haemorrhages may develop. After two days follicles appear on the palpebral conjunctiva but the follicular response is varied. Pseudomembrane formation in some cases and marked edema of conjunctival tissue may mask the follicular changes. At this stage preauricular and even cervical lymphadenopathy is usually present in about half of patients. Lymphnode enlargement and tenderness is variable, but more prominant on the side of the eye first involved in bilateral disease. (Laibson, 1975). In most patients the enlarged lymphnodes gradually diminish to disappear in the first two weeks.

During the first week *corneal changes* in the form of diffuse superficial keratitis begin to manifest. According to Laibson (1975), early fine diffuse punctate keratitis may be easily missed unless biomicroscopy is done with retroillumination or side illumination. The diffuse keratitis does not stain with fluorescein or rose bengal and cannot be detected by slit beam or direct illumination. In the second week the fine epithelial keratitis changes to ground glass type focal lesions of corneal epithelium with increase in pain, lacrimation, photophobia and visual disturbances. Blepharospasm may ensue. Focal spots of keratitis are larger than punctate lesions and stain with fluorescein and rose bengal. They vary in shape, size and number. The focal lesions are commonly located in the center of the cornea (fig. VII-3), but may be scattered all over the cornea or involve only the limbal area. Gradually, subepithelial infiltrates develop under the focal superficial lesions. In the third week these infiltrates may have become entirely subepithelial.

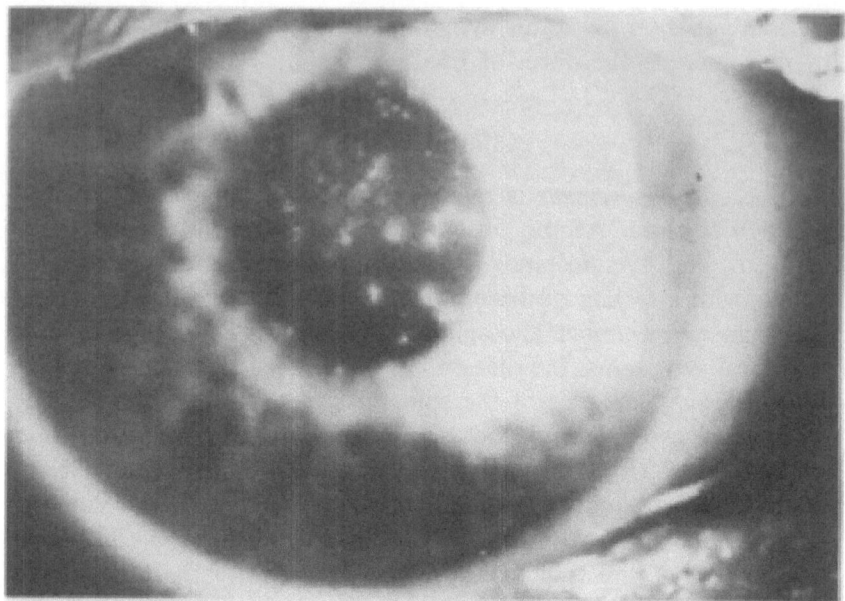

Fig. VII-3. — Coarse punctate lesions mostly involving central cornea in EKC.

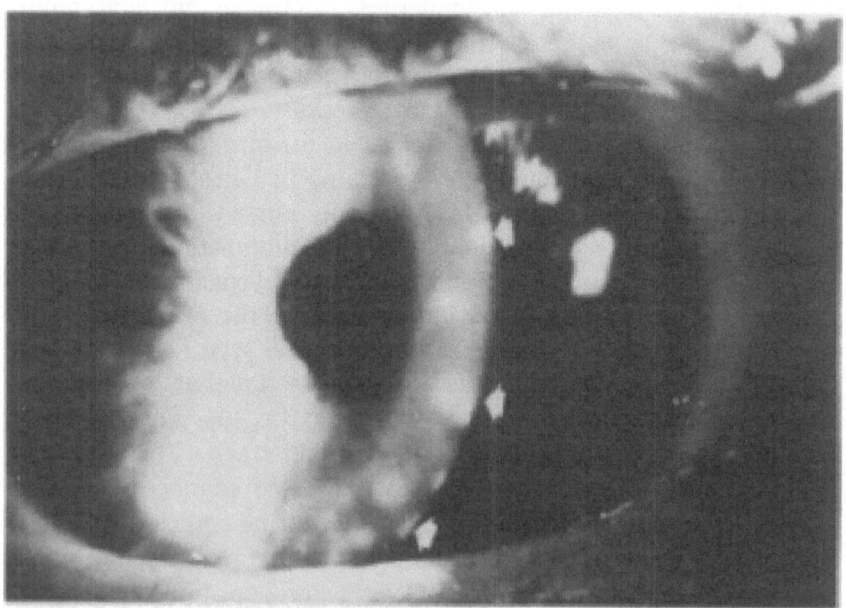

Fig. VII-4. — Discoid subepithelial opacities (arrows) in EKC after the epithelial component of the disease is healed.

As the epithelial disease disappears typical subepithelial opacities are located beneath the Bowman's membrane (fig. VII-4). Sometimes, however, deep stromal opacities develop. Like the focal epithelial lesions, the number, size, shape, and the location of subepithelial opacities is variable. When discoid in appearance they resemble lesions of nummular keratitis. The overlying epithelium no longer stains with vital dyes. The subepithelial opacities gradually fade and disappear over several months to more than 2 years. Rarely, sharp bordered stromal scars may develop. The nature of the subepithelial opacities is not well known. However, they appear to be secondary reaction to the epithelial lesions. One may assume that they consist of precipitated immune complexes, invaded by leucocytes attracted by chemotaxis. The presence of leucocytes may explain why the overlying epithelial cells remain abnormal for a long period when adenovirus is no longer present in the epithelium. The above mentioned hypothesis would also explain why early removal of the epithelium by an abrasion or replica prevents the formation of subepithelial opacities. The effect of cortisone on the reduction of these opacities is also explained by this hypothesis.

Occasionally the clinical picture may differ from classical disease. Severe keratitis with corneal edema, folds in Descemet's membrane, endothelitis and anterior uveitis may develop. Large epithelial erosions are seen in a small number of patients. Our limited observations are in agreement with Laibson (1975) that in such eyes after healing, surprisingly, very few subepithelial infiltrates develop, if at all. Symblepharon formation is a rare complication of EKC. Boniuk et al. (1966) described unusual cases of adenovirus keratoconjunctivitis. In one patient a sector shaped diffuse epithelial lesion due to type 2 adenovirus persisted for nearly two years in the absence of follicular conjunctivitis and despite epithelium debridement. Another patient suffered from recurrent keratoconjunctivitis of 1 to 2 weeks duration with intervening asymptomatic periods. Type 3 adenovirus was isolated from the eye.

Pathology

Duke-Elder (1965) reviewed the *histological studies* of EKC. Degenerative changes in stroma with infiltration of mononuclear cells and some polymorphonuclear leukocytes occurs at the site of lesions. Bowman's membrane is thinned or even interrupted. The stromal

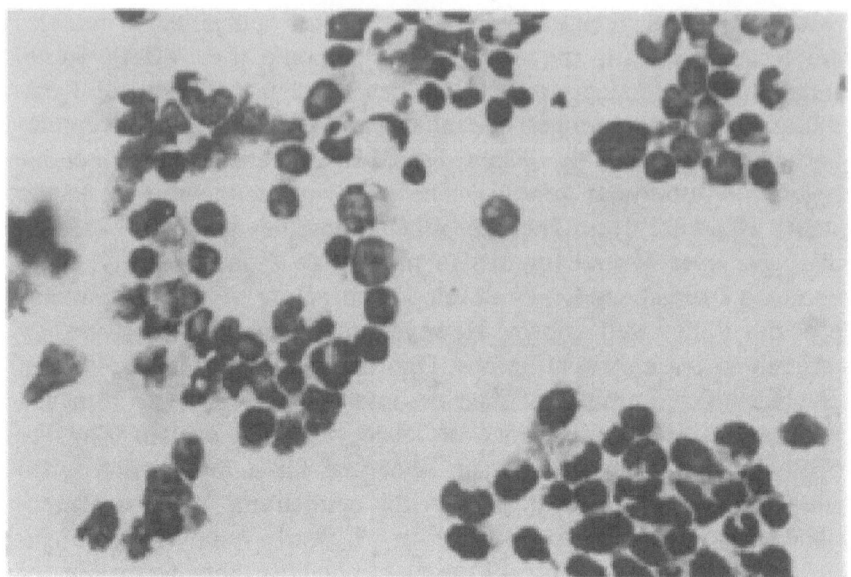

Fig. VII-5. — Predominant mononuclear cell response in conjunctival scraping from a patient of EKC in the early acute stage. Giemsa stain. ×660.

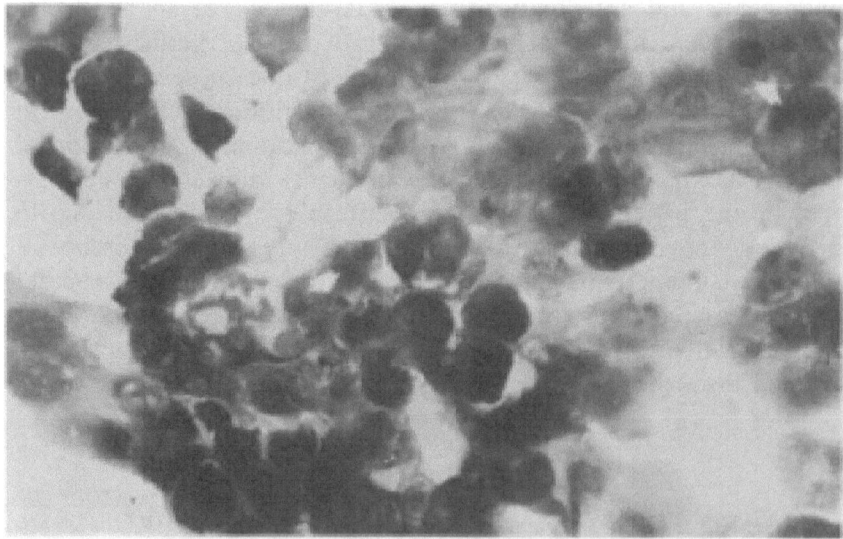

Fig. VII-6. — Flat mount of cells by corneal replica technique shows cell degeneration and rounding of superficial cells in the epithelial lesion of EKC. Variable sized rounded inclusions (arrows) are seen in the degenerating cells. Hematoxylin-eosin stain. ×800.

changes appear to result from antigen-antibody reaction. Intranuclear inclusion bodies may be detected in Giemsa stained corneal and conjunctival scrapings (Boniuk et al., 1966) which also show abundant mononuclear cells (fig. VII-5). The study of corneal replicas shows plasma membrane alterations, cell rounding, degeneration and rounded inclusion bodies during the early stage of epithelial keratitis (fig. VII-6). Electron microscopy may reveal adenovirus in the cells of conjunctival and corneal epithelium (Segawa, 1962). The conjunctival pseudomembrane is formed of fibrin with mononuclear and polymorphonuclear leukocyte infiltration (Laibson and Green, 1970; Dawson et al., 1972).

Diagnostic laboratory investigations

Fluorescein labelled specific antibody binds to the infected epithelium cells in scrapings. Direct and indirect immunofluorescence techniques are available for this purpose (Uchida and Inove, 1967; Inove, 1968, 1971; Ishizu, 1969; Vastine et al., 1977). Virus isolation from the eye and determination of rising serum antibody titers are in current use to establish the diagnosis of EKC. Adenovirus can be isolated in about 80% of cases from conjunctival swabbings and scrapings during the first 10 days of disease (Ellison et al., 1969). During convalescence, significant rise in complement fixing and specific virus neutralizing antibodies is found. In the early acute phase serum should be checked for the normal level of antibodies found in each patient. Maximum antibody titers occur about 2 to 3 weeks after infection, which gradually decline but may persist for a year or longer (Locatcher-Khorazo and Seegal, 1972). A four fold rise or fall in antibody titers taken at acute, convalescent or late stages of disease is considered confirmatory of adenovirus infection.

Treatment

No specific *treatment* is available. Use of topical corticosteroids may delay the development of corneal opacities, which reappear on the withdrawal of treatment (Laibson et al., 1970; Dawson et al., 1972; Freyler and Sehorst, 1976). Antiviral agents, IDU and Ara-A, are ineffective in EKC (Hecht et al., 1965; Dudgeon et al., 1969; Pavan-Langston and Dohlman, 1972; and Warring et al., 1976). Wassileva and Galabov (1975) reported that ABOB (1', 1'-anhydrobis (2-hydroxy-ethyl) biguanide) (Virustat®) 1%, when topically applied reduced the severity of keratitis and suppressed the development of corneal opacities in treated patients in an open study. In a limited number of patients we observed prompt healing of epithelial lesions, both punctate focal spots and large erosions, after making a corneal replica. No subepithelial opacities developed after the replica procedure.

CHLAMYDIAL KERATOCONJUNCTIVITIS

Chlamydia agents were considered to be large viruses, but they are more closely related to bacteria since they possess both DNA and RNA and some enzyme systems. Moreover, they divide by binary fission, are sensitive to some antibiotics and sulfonamides and possess a cell wall containing muramic acid (Perkins and Ellison, 1963; Sarov and Becker, 1963; Bietti and Werner, 1967; Sarov and Becker, 1968; 1971a and 1971b; and Gutter and Becker, 1972).

The trachoma agent (C-trachomatis) was isolated only in 1957 by Chinese workers (Tang et al., 1957), even though Halberstaedter and von Prowazek (1907) had described typical cytoplasmic inclusions fifty years earlier.

The various chlamydia agents are similar in morphology. The smallest infectious particle, the elementary body, measures 0.2 to 0.3 mμ in diameter (Thygeson et al., 1935). The larger initial bodies vary in size, upto 0.7μ, and are much less infectious. Upon release by cell bursting, the elementary bodies infect other cells.

Although chlamydia have a common group antigen, they are divided into subgroup A (C-trachomatis) and subgroup B (C-psittaci). C-trachomatis includes the agents producing trachoma, inclusion conjunctivitis, and lymphogranuloma venereum. C-psittaci includes the agents responsible for psittacosis, bovine abortion, feline pneumonitis and some other infections in animals and birds (Dawson, 1975). The inclusion bodies of C-trachomatis are rigid and compact; they contain glycogen and are inhibited by sulfonamides and some antibiotics. On the contrary, the C-psittaci are resistant to the action of sulfonamides and antibiotics; their inclusions are irregular and flexible, and do not possess glycogen in the matrix.

The oculogenital and genital diseases produced by C-trachomatis are classified in table VII-2. The term "TRIC" includes the agents producing trachoma (TR) and inclusion conjunctivitis (IC) in man.

TABLE VII-2. — *Oculogenital diseases caused by C-trachomatis*

Oculogenital	Genital
Trachoma	Lymphogranuloma venereum
Ophthalmia neonatorum	Urethritis both in males and females
Inclusion conjunctivitis	Cervicitis
TRIC punctate keratoconjunctivitis	Salpingitis (in females)
	Abortion
	Reiters' disease (?)
	Proctitis

C-trachomatis is further divided into different serotypes on the basis of microtiter indirect immunofluorescent test. Serotypes A, B, Ba, and C have been isolated from the eyes of trachoma patients in endemic areas (McComb and Nichols, 1970; Hanna et al., 1973; Briones et al., 1974; Wang and Grayston, 1974; Dawson, 1975) while serotypes D, E, F, G, H, I, J, and K and sometimes B and C cause ophthalmia neonatorum, adult inclusion conjunctivitis and genital tract infections (McComb and Nichols, 1970; Wang et al., 1973; Wang and Grayston, 1974; Dawson, 1975). Some authors restrict the term C-trachomatis to the serotypes causing trachoma while the serotypes causing ocular and genital disease are grouped under C-oculogenitalis (Thygeson, 1971; Grayson, 1979).

TRACHOMA

Trachoma "is a specific communicable kerato-conjunctivitis, usually of chronic evolution caused by the chlamydia trachomatis, primarily affecting the superficial epithelium, characterized by the formation of follicles, papillary hyperplasia and pannus; the natural resolution of which is by cicatrization, involving potentially considerable visual disability" (Duke-Elder, 1965).

Duke-Elder (1965) has also reviewed the history of trachoma which dates back to the earliest medical records upto 27th Century B.C. in China.

Epidemiology

According to surveys of Bietti et al. (1962) and Bietti and Werner (1967), trachoma is endemic in large parts of the world. At present, Belgium is one of the few countries where it is practically extinct (almost all cases are foreign immigrants or Belgians returning after prolonged stay in endemic areas). However, no race is immune from trachoma but some are more susceptible than others. The number of trachomatous patients throughout the world has been estimated from 400 to 500 million (Bietti, 1972).

Trachoma is commonly transmitted from eye to eye by contact with contaminated hands (Jones et al., 1976). The disease spreads in overcrowded communities living under poor hygienic conditions. Flies, contaminated towels, bed-clothes or other fomites also play an important role in the spread of trachoma in hyperendemic areas. Poverty and social customs opposed to personal hygiene are two important obstacles in the battle against this disease.

Pathogenesis

The pathogenesis of trachoma is not well understood. In histological (Duke-Elder, 1965) and electron-microscopic (Mitsui and Suzuki, 1965) studies C-trachomatis has been detected only in the epithelial cells of the cornea and conjunctiva. Furthermore, transcutaneous injection of infective material into the subepithelial tissues of the lids does not produce disease. As a consequence, the production of a soluble and diffusible toxin is thought to be responsible for the gross subepithelial lymphoid response and subsequent scarring (Duke-Elder, 1965; Silverstein, 1974).

Pathology

Extensive histological studies on trachoma have been done. We shall consider here the important histopathological features. For a detailed description the reader should refer to System of Ophthalmology, Vol. VIII, Part I by Duke-Elder (1965), from where the following account has largerly been drawn.

During the early stage of the disease characteristic Halberstaedter-Prowazek cytoplasmic inclusions are found in the conjunctival and corneal epithelium. In Giemsa stained scrapings or smears, the elementary bodies appear red to purple while the initial bodies are blue. In the chronic and cicatricial stages they are only infrequently seen. Associated histological features may help in the diagnosis of trachoma in the absence of typical inclusion bodies. These include: abundant polymorphonuclear neutrophils, small and medium sized lymphocytes, plasma cells, blastoid cells and other stem cells, Leber cells

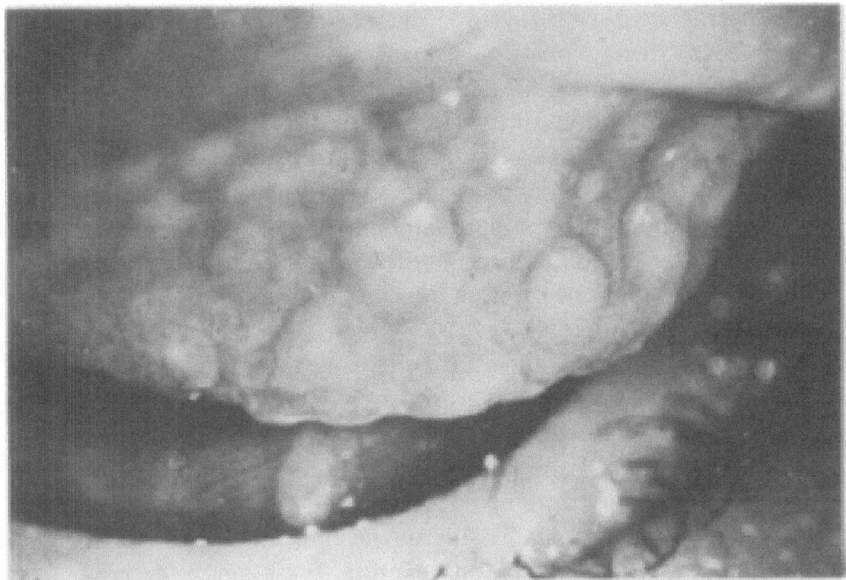

Fig. VII-7. — Large sagograin-like follicles on the upper eyelid in stage II trachoma.

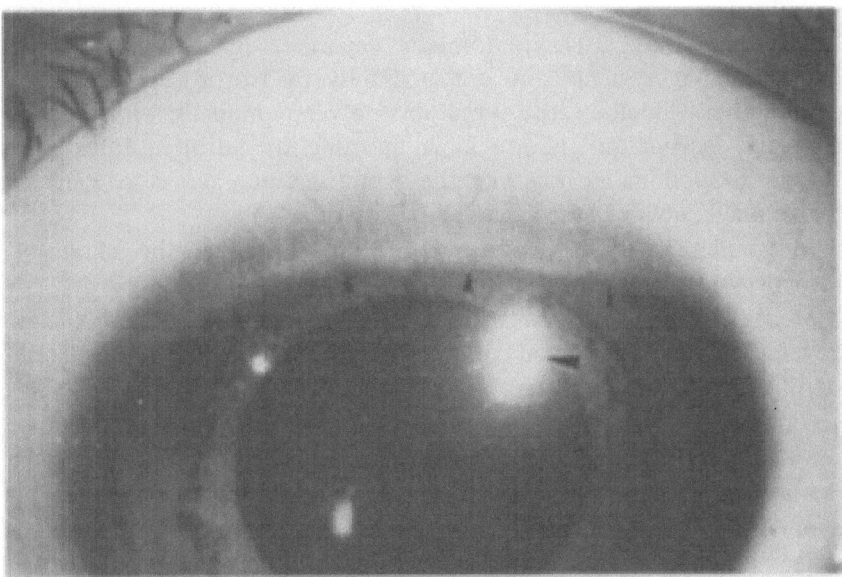

Fig. VII-8. — Trachomatous pannus (small arrows). Scattered light reflex on the cornea denotes the surface irregularities (large arrow).

(large macrophages with ingested cytoplasmic debris), and the multinucleated epithelial cells.

Hypertrophic changes of the epithelium occur at the same time with papillae formation. Infiltration of many lymphocytes, plasma cells and some mononuclear leukocytes and histiocytes, leads to follicular hypertrophy. Eosinophiles and mast cells are present deep in the tissues. Among the cellular elements connective tissue fibers are found which by proliferation produce characteristic cicatrization. With the progression of disease, degeneration and necrosis occurs in the center of the follicles.

Infiltration of tarsus and subsequent degeneration produces lid deformities. Bulbar conjunctiva only infrequently shows true follicle formation.

Diffuse hazyness of the corneal epithelium and multiple punctate erosions progress to combined epithelial and subepithelial keratitis. Vascular invasion from the limbus accompanied by lymphocytic infiltration leads to trachomatous pannus formation.

Lacrimal gland involvement is infrequent but occlusion of the lacrimal ductules commonly occurs.

Clinical picture

Trachoma may be asymptomatic, especially in individuals with good personal hygiene, and detected only by scarring of the tarsal conjunctiva. Generally, the symptoms develop gradually with moderate pain, lacrimation, photophobia and slightly purulent thick discharge. Exceptionally, however, the symptoms may be acute. Pannus formation is always associated with irritation.

MacCallan in 1936 (Duke-Elder, 1965) classified the clinically recognizable disease into four stages:

Stage I. After an incubation period of 5 to 12 days, follicles develop on the upper tarsal conjunctiva due to lymphoid hyperplasia. A diffuse punctate keratitis, best observed by biomicroscopy, usually accompanies. This early stage may persist for 3 months to 3 years.

Stage II a. The tarsal conjunctiva becomes swollen with large sagograin like follicles (fig. VII-7). These follicles are soft and easily expressible, a feature that distinguishes them from the follicles in other diseases. Keratitis progresses further and becomes visible without magnification. Pannus formation is the rule and limbal follicles may be present (fig. VII-8).

Halberstaedter-Prowazek inclusion bodies are detected in the scrapings obtained in stages I and IIa.

The stage IIa lasts from 3 months to 3 years.

Stage IIb. If secondary bacterial infection occurs or in some cases of highly virulent trachoma, follicular change may be marked by papillary hypotrophy. It may progress into stage III or regress into stage IIa.

Stage III. Cicatrization occurs during this stage, accompanied by progressive decrease in the activity of inflammation. This phase may last for several years.

Stage IV. The disease is no longer active. Follicles on the tarsus are replaced by connective tissue (fig. VII-9). Cicatrization of limbal follicles leads to peripheral Herbert's pits. Shrinkage of conjunctiva may occur resulting in trichiasis and enteropion. Obliteration of lacrimal ductules may produce dry eye. Extensive pannus formation (fig. VII-10) and scarring, when present, severely reduce visual acuity.

Trachomatous ptosis or the typical drooping of the upper eyelid (fig. VII-11) is present from the initial stages of the disease. It is caused in part by the swollen lids and in part due to the infiltration of Müllers muscle.

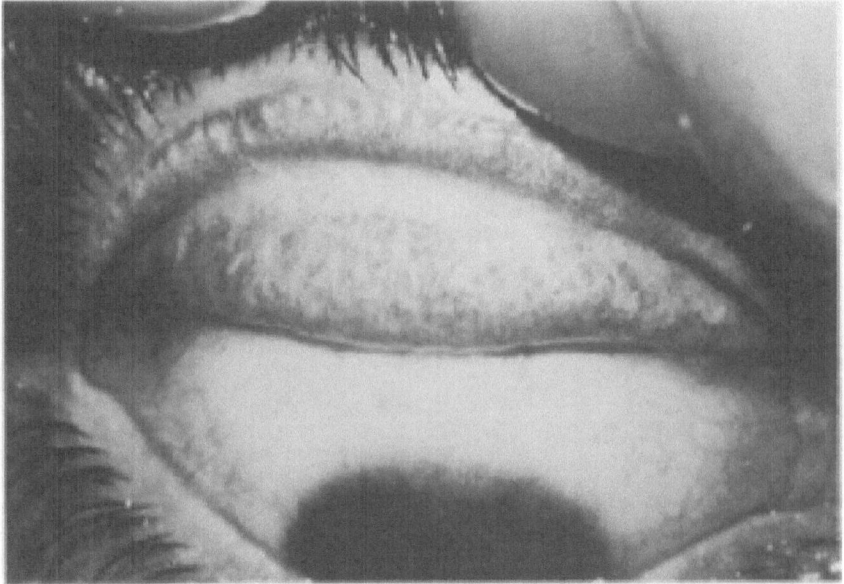

Fig. VII-9. — Typical scarring of the upper tarsus in trachoma. Note a small pannus.

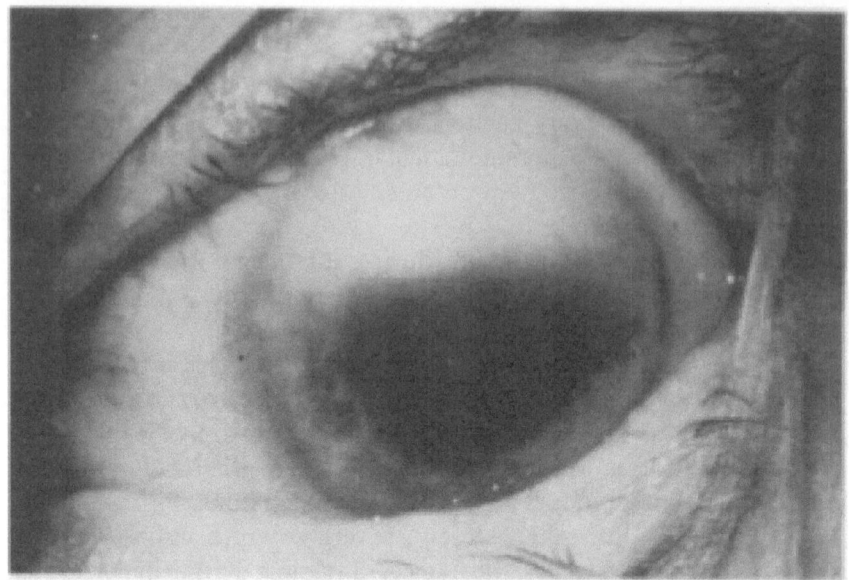

Fig. VII-10. — Extensive pannus formation in trachoma.

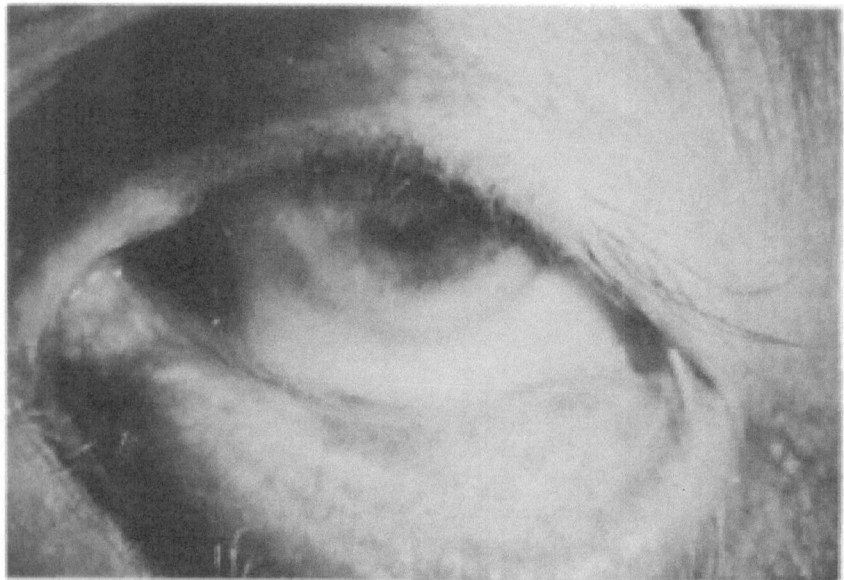

Fig. VII-11. — Drooping of the upper eyelid gives a typical sleepy appearance. (The lower eyelid was everted before photography).

The clinical course and prognosis are extremely variable. The disease may remain mild or spontaneous cure may occur in the absence of bacterial superinfections. In other cases chronic course resistant to treatment is seen.

Diagnosis

Diagnosis in the early stages may be difficult, if one is not acquainted with the disease, as other types of conjunctivitis may simulate trachoma. However, the development of early follicles on the conjunctiva or limbus, superficial keratitis involving the upper part of the cornea, trachomatous pannus most pronounced around the superior limbus, and typical cicatrization of the upper tarsal conjunctiva are typical distinguishing features of this disease. According to the World Health Organization report (1962), at least two of the following signs should be present for the diagnosis of trachoma:

1. Lymphoid follicles on the upper tarsal conjunctiva, limbal follicles or their sequelae.
2. Epithelial or subepithelial keratitis, especially on the upper third of the cornea.
3. Pannus in the upper part of the cornea.
4. Typical scars.

Detection of inclusion bodies in the Giemsa and iodine staining is confirmatory of trachoma. Other cytological features like polymorphonuclear neutrophils, lymphocytes, eosinophils, plasma cells, blast cells, Leber cells, and multinucleated epithelial cells are indicative of chlamydia infection (Yoneda et al., 1975). The scrapings may also be stained by the fluorescent antibody staining techniques. Isolation of chlamydia trachomatis may be done in the yolk sac of embryonated eggs (Tang et al., 1957) or in irradiated tissue culture cell systems (Gordon and Quan, 1965). Finally, an infection with chlamydia agents can be detected by serological methods, i.e. complement fixation test and microtiter indirect immunofluorescent test. Detection of serum antibodies indicates infection in the past. During the active disease the antibody titers are raised.

INCLUSION CONJUNCTIVITIS

Inclusion conjunctivitis is a venerally transmitted relatively benign follicular conjunctivitis caused by C-oculogenitalis. Two clinical forms are recognised: *inclusion blenorrhea in the new born,* and *inclusion conjunctivitis in older children and adults.*

Inclusion blenorrhea (chlamydial infection) may occur in 3% of all new born babies in U.S.A. (Grayson, 1979). The infection is acquired during birth from mother's infected birth canal (Thygeson, 1971). It manifests as a papillary conjunctivitis with profuse mucopurulent discharge after 5-12 days (Locatcher-Khorazo and Seegal, 1972; Ostler, 1976; Grayson, 1979). Neither follicles nor preauricular lymphadenopathy occurs in the newborn. Follicles may appear after 6 weeks. Infrequently, conjunctival pseudomembranes form which always result in mild scarring (Hansman, 1969; Forster et al., 1970). *Corneal involvement* is generally limited to a fine epithelial keratitis but micropannus, stromal haze and infiltrates may develop (Grayson, 1979).

The disease is usually self-limited, resolving spontaneously in 2-4 weeks or longer. A longer course, if left untreated, will produce a higher incidence of micropannus and stromal scarring. Forster et al. (1970) found micropannus and mild conjunctival scarring in six of nine children, 7 months to 11 years later. Persistent TRIC infection was demonstrated by immunofluorescent technique in one 7 year old child.

Inclusion conjunctivitis of older children and adults is an oculogenital disease marked by follicular conjunctivitis, mucopurulent discharge, photophobia and irridation. C-oculogenitalis affects the conjunctiva and genito-urinary epithelia, and may persist in these sites for years forming a potential source of ocular reinfection (Havener, 1978). Infection spreads from genitalia to the eyes by contaminated fingers or fomites.

The disease develops after 3 to 4 days of exposure, is frequently unilateral and becomes bilateral after 2 to 3 weeks (Duke-Elder, 1965). Initially, the palpebral conjunctiva is diffusely red and swollen. Preauricular lymphnodes are enlarged but non-tender. After about a week conjunctival follicles appear. The lower lid is more severely involved than the upper. Cornea may show epithelial keratitis and micropannus formation. Spontaneous resolution is slow and gradual, taking from 6 months to more than a year.

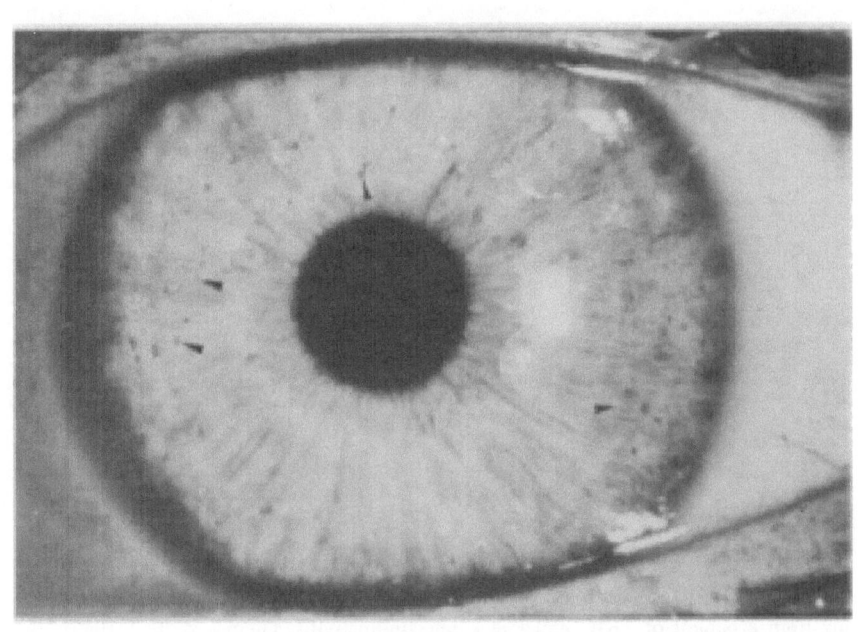

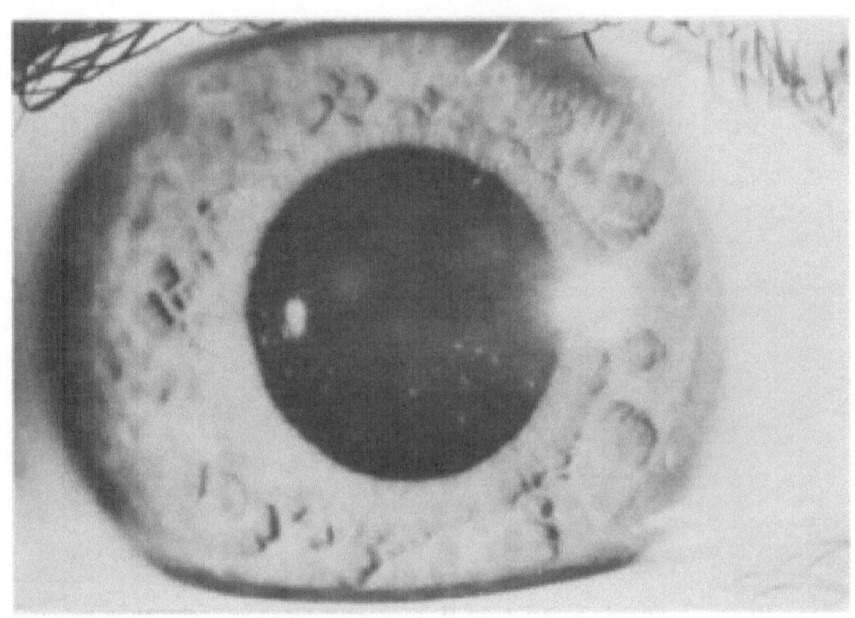

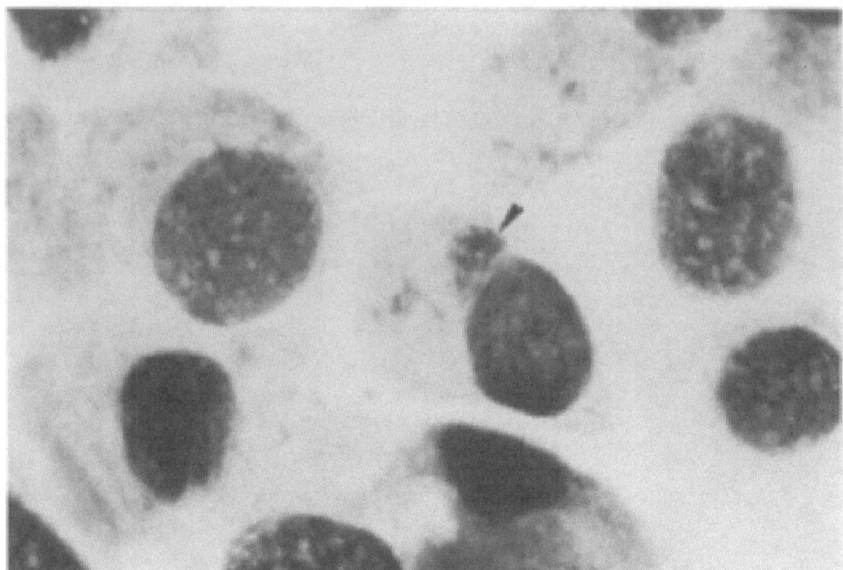

Fig. VII-14. — Halberstaedter-Prowazec inclusion (arrow) in the conjunctival scraping from a patient of TRIC punctate keratoconjunctivitis. Giemsa stain. × 1050.

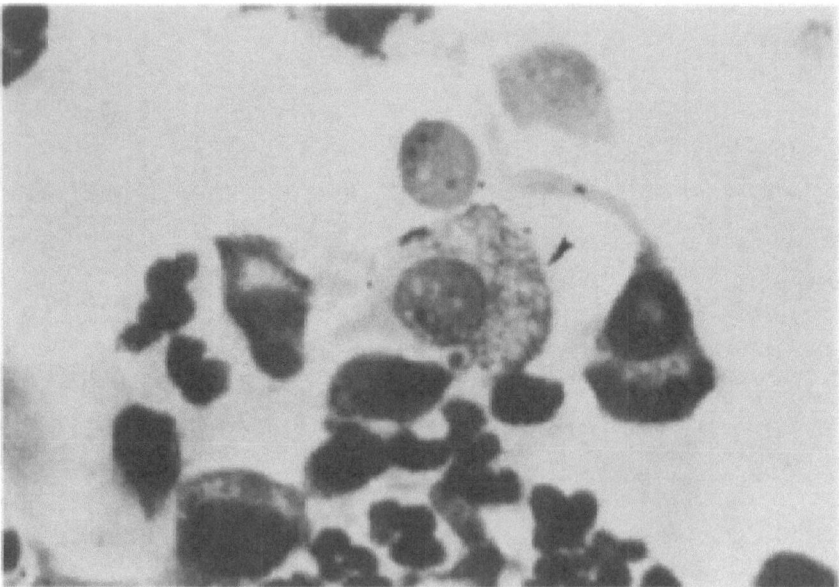

Fig. VII-15. — Loosely packed large Halberstaedter-Prowazec inclusion in the cytoplasm of a cell (arrow) in the conjunctival scraping. Adult inclusion conjunctivitis. Giemsa stain. × 810.

TRIC punctate keratoconjunctivitis. This condition is a typical inclusion conjunctivitis accompanied by punctate epithelial and subepithelial keratitis (figs. VII-12 and VII-13). Duke-Elder (1965) describes it as a clinical syndrome intermediate between typical trachoma and inclusion conjunctivitis. Subepithelial infiltrates develop under the epithelial lesions which persist after the epithelial component is healed. Successive crops of lesions may develop upto about one year followed by a chronic healing stage.

Laboratory diagnostic methods of inclusion conjunctivitis in adult and newborn are samilar to those used for the identification of trachoma. Figures VII-14 and VII-15 show typical Halberstaedter-Prowazek inclusion bodies.

Treatment of chlamydia infections

Chlamydial oculogenital disease responds to local and systemic sulfonamides and some antibiotics like tetracyclines, erythromycin, penicillin (Havener, 1978), although the sensitivity of various agents may differ. Generally, continued topical therapy from 2 to 6 weeks suffices, but sometimes may have to be continued for 3 months or longer. As the urogenital epithelia are the source of infection; inclusion conjunctivitis should be treated by oral sulfonamides or tetracyclines. The affected family members or the sexual contacts of the patient should be treated at the same time to prevent re-infections.

In its early stage trachoma responds well to topical antibiotic therapy. However, in endemic areas re-infections usually occur. The treatment in the late cicatricial stages is mainly surgical.

THYGESON'S SUPERFICIAL PUNCTATE KERATITIS

Thygeson (1950) described a bilateral superficial coarse punctate keratitis without conjunctivitis, characterized by multiple punctate epithelial lesions and prolonged course with remissions and exacerbations. It is a well defined clinical entity of obscure etiology. Although three decades have elapsed since Thygeson's initial description, only a few reports have appeared in literature, probably because of misdiagnosis and confusion with other types of keratitis.

Epidemiology

According to Thygeson (1950; 1961 and 1966), this type of keratitis occurs all over the United States. It has also been reported in England, France, West Germany, Iran, Senegal and Ivory coast. (Braley, 1950; Braley and Alexander, 1953; Jones, 1960 and 1963; Brini and Payeur, 1966; Quéré et al., 1967, 1968 and 1973; Sundmacher, 1976 and 1977; Pirouz, 1977).

Both sexes are equally affected and the disease has been reported at all ages except in infants. All reported cases are sporadic. It does not spread among the close contacts and family members. There are no associated systemic symptoms.

Etiology

The cause of Thygeson's superficial punctate keratitis is unknown. Braley and Alexander (1953) reported to have isolated a virus from the corneal epithelium, but it has not been confirmed. Recently, Lemp et al. (1974) isolated herpes zoster virus from the eye of a patient with superficial punctate keratitis, but the authors themselves wondered if it was a chance discovery. We detected yeast-like bodies in the punctate lesions by replica technique in three clinically typical cases of Thygeson's keratitis (unpublished). However, at this stage, we are unable to say if the yeast infections are the cause of punctate keratitis or merely a superinfection.

Since the disease is not contagious and responds well to topical corticosteroids, an allergic etiology is envisaged but not proven; although 8 of 28 patients in one serie had some allergic disorders (Quéré et al., 1973).

Jones (1963) suggested that Thygeson's superficial punctate keratitis may represent an epithelial dystrophy.

Clinical picture

Both eyes are affected in most cases but symptoms may be more pronounced in one eye. Only one case has been reported with unilateral disease (Quéré et al., 1968).

The symptoms are persistent and annoying. During an exacerbation there is burning, irritation, foreign body sensation, lacrimation and intense photophobia. We have seen four cases of Thygeson's keratitis during the last 3 years. All of them wore dark glasses even on cloudy days. One patient was a 5 year old girl who did not want to open her eyes in the morning as it " pained " on doing so. Because of photophobia it was difficult to examine these patients on slit-lamp. Photophobia was much more pronounced than in other cases of keratitis.

The symptoms are aggravated by visual effort and activities demanding prolonged concentration. Ocular discomfort and lacrimation increased in our patients while testing the visual acuity. Activities like sewing, reading, watching television etc. may not be possible, as all of them aggravate the symptoms (Quéré et al., 1968).

On examination there is no mucoid secretion in the eye. Vision may be slightly reduced. The cornea shows variable number (average 20 to 25) of coarse punctate epithelial opacities, usually located in the center, but may involve any part of the cornea, or be diffusely scattered all over its surface (fig. VII-16). The punctate lesions are rounded or oval but may assume stellate or irregular form. Each lesion is a collection of fine grey dots slightly raised above the epithelial surface and staining intensely with rose bengal, moderately with fluorescein, and feebly with methylene blue (Quéré et al., 1973). The punctate lesions vary in size. They start as a fine punctate lesion

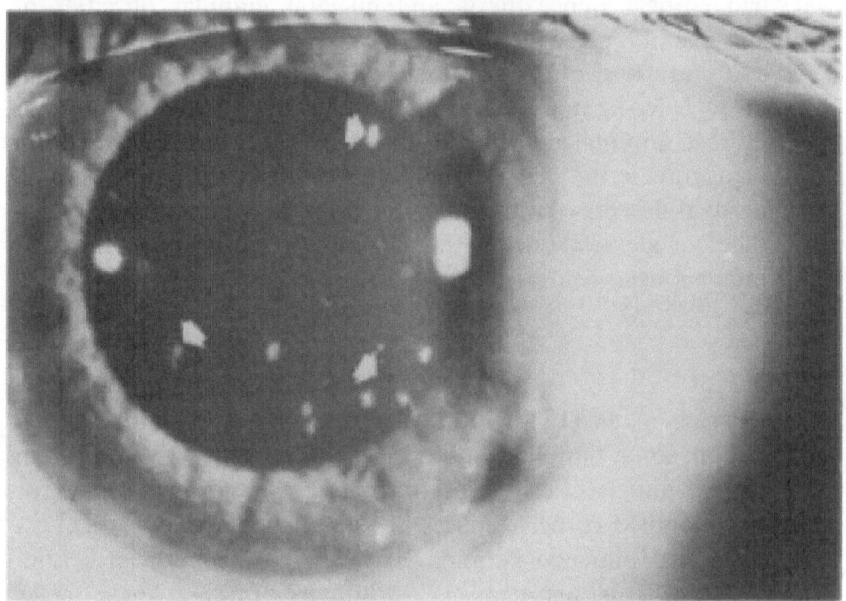

Fig. VII-16. — Thygeson's superficial punctate keratitis. Some of the epithelial lesions are indicated by arrows.

which gradually enlarges. Decrease in size and healing follows after central desquamation (Braley and Alexander, 1953). The stroma remains uninvolved, excepting some edematous changes under the lesions. The corneal area free of punctate lesions clinically appears normal. While the existing lesions heal in an average period of 3 to 8 days, new ones appear. Sometimes, filaments may form (Braley and Alexander, 1953).

Generally, the eyes are white but the bulbar conjunctiva may be hyperemic. The corneal sensitivity is normal. The palpebral conjunctiva is normal and there is no regional lymphadenopathy. There are no associated systemic symptoms or disease. No complications have been reported and healing occurs without sequelae.

The clinical course is characterized by remissions and exacerbations over a long period, extending from 6 months to 10 years, but on the average 2 to 4 years. During remission the eye is white and the corneal epithelium may be normal, but usually a few corneal punctate lesions are present. According to Quéré et al. (1968) a very short stay on the beach or exposure to cigarette smoke may provoke the signs and symptoms. Another patient suffered an exacerbation after the week-ends when he had been on safari. This patient, however, had corneal hypoesthesia and bilateral granular opacities of Bowman's membrane, which make the diagnosis of Thygeson's keratitis doubtful. Regarding the first two cases, it is possible that exposure to U.V.-light on beach and smoke may irritate the eye or have a direct minimal detrimental effect on the corneal epithelium, and thus aggravate the ocular condition. One of our patients suffered from the recrudescence of disease after he rode a motor-cycle, without protective glasses, during the healing phase. A mosquito had fallen into his eye.

Pathology

Sundmacher et al. (1977) found various degrees of epithelial cell degeneration, some lymphocyte-like cells and secondary lysosomes in the epithelial punctate lesions by transmission electron microscopy.

We have studied corneal replicas of three patients showing Thygeson's superficial punctate keratitis. The whole of superficial epithelium shows edematous changes, although clinically these areas appear normal. The punctate lesions vary in size and possess irregular borders. There is no palisading of elongated cells around the

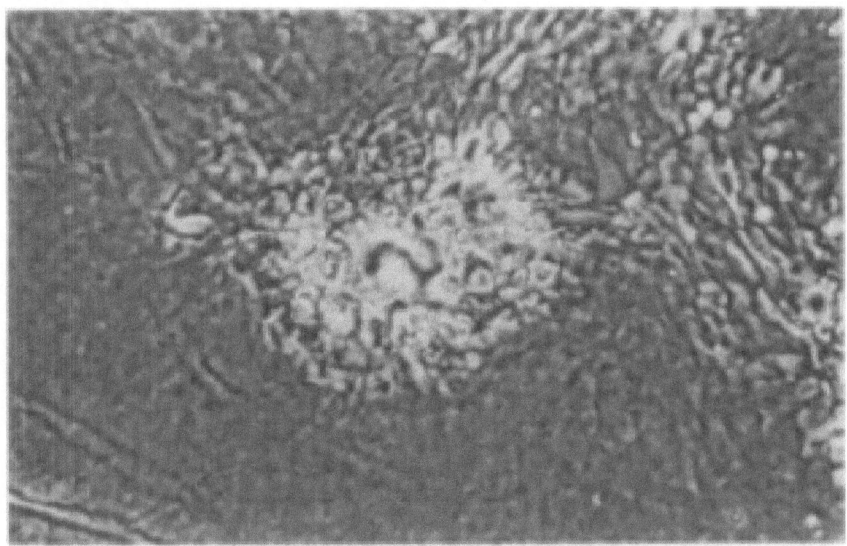

Fig. VII-17. — Corneal replica shows necrosis and rounding of the cells in the punctate lesions of Thygeson's keratitis. Phase contrast microscopy. × 330.

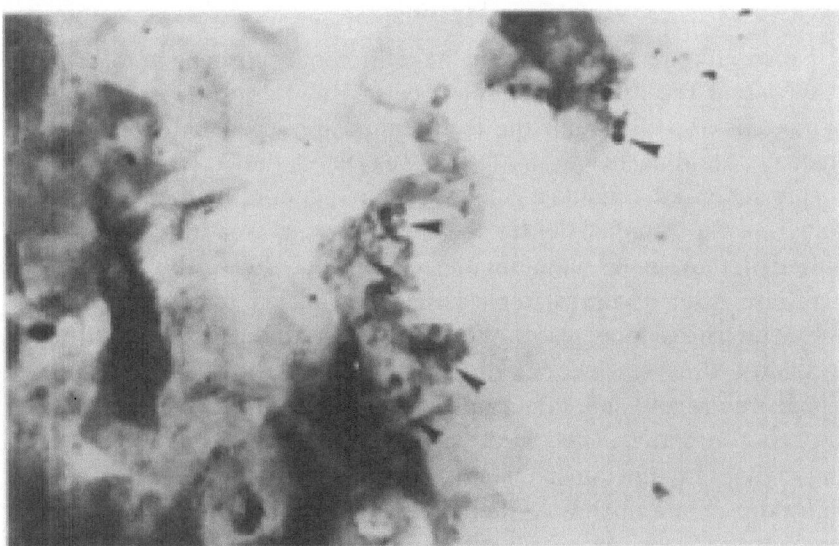

Fig. VII-18. — Yeast-like bodies (arrows) in Thygeson's superficial punctate keratitis. Giemsa stain. × 810.

lesions like that seen in the herpes simplex punctate keratitis (fig. VII-17). The small lesions are made of edematous or rounded cells. The small punctate spots probably represent the early new lesions or the old healing lesions. The larger lesions contained degenerated and necrosed cells in the center, some of them fusing together. These cells were alcian blue positive in the combined alcian blue-PAS staining, while the surrounding edematous cells gave a positive PAS reaction. Yeast-like bodies were identified in the lesions (fig. VII-18). They stained violet with alcian blue and PAS stain. Similar structures were also detected in the corneal replicas of two other patients of Thygeson's keratitis, associated with bacterial infection. In a fourth patient conjunctival scrapings contained yeast bodies.

Since yeast or candida are widespread naturally occurring microorganisms, their detection in the corneal replicas of these patients could be a superinfection. However, we have not found similar structures in nearly hundred replicas of patients having viral, bacterial, fungal or non specific keratitis. Since the clinical picture and the course of disease in our patients was typical of Thygeson's superficial punctate keratitis, our findings suggest that yeast infection could be the etiological factor in this disease. However, further studies are required to clarify the role of yeast infections in Thygeson's keratitis.

Treatment

No specific treatment is available. Different reports have repeatedly emphasized the efficacy of topical corticosteroids in suppressing the symptoms and signs, but the recurrences may occur on stopping the therapy. Sundmacher et al. (1977) suggested the alternative use of highly hydrophilic contact lenses. In our patients neither corticosteroids nor soft contact lenses were effective in treating the disease, although they gave symptomatic relief and reduced the severity of keratitis. After a corneal replica the eyes healed temporarily before the recurrences took place. We treated our three patients with 1% nystatin or flucystosine, one drop instilled every hour during the day. There was remarkable effect on the symptoms. Two patients healed within 4 months. The third patient was lost to follow-up while improving. In the fourth patient, who also had associated bacterial infection, chloramphenicol therapy lead to healing in two weeks.

BIBLIOGRAPHY

Béal, R. — Sur une forme particulière de conjunctivite aigue avec des follicules. *Ann. Oculist.*, *87*, 1, 1907.

Bell, J.A., Rowe, W.P., Engler, J.I., Parrott, R.H. and Huebner, R.J. — Pharyngoconjunctival fever, epidemiological studies of a recently recognized disease entity. *J.A.M.A.*, *157*, 1083, 1955.

Bell, J.A., Ward, R.G., Huebner, R.J., Rowe, W.P., Suskind, R.G. and Paffenbarger, R.S. — Studies of adenoviruses (APC) in volunteers. *Amer. J. Public Health*, *46*, 1130, 1956.

Bell, J.A. — Epidemiology of pharyngoconjunctival fever. *Amer. J. Ophthal.*, *43*, 36, 1957.

Bietti, G.B. and Bruna, F. — Epidemic keratoconjunctivitis in Italy. Some contributions to its clinical aspects, epidemiology and etiology. *Amer. J. Ophthal.*, *43*, 50, 1957.

Bietti, G.B., Freyche, M.J. and Vozza, R. — La diffusion actuelle du trachome dans le monde. *Rev. Int. Trachome*, *39*, 113, 1962.

Bietti, G.B. and Werner, G.H. — In: *Trachoma: Prevention and treatment*. Kugelmass, I.N. Ed. Charles C. Thomas, — Springfield, 1967.

Bietti, G.B. — Natural history and diagnosis of trachoma. *Israel J. Med. Sci.*, *8*, 1101, 1972.

Boni, B.M. and Schmidt, N. — Self-induced epidemic keratoconjunctivitis. *J.A.M.A.*, *238*, 396, 1977.

Boniuk, M., Phillips, C.A., Hines, M.J. and Friedman, J.B. — Adenovirus infections of the conjunctiva and cornea. *Trans. Am. Acad. Ophthal. Otolaryng.*, *70*, 1016, 1966.

Braley, A.E. — Virus disease of the cornea. *Med. Res. (Houston)*, *44*, 102, 1950.

Braley, A.E. and Alexander, R.C. — Superficial punctate keratitis (isolation of a virus). *Arch. Ophthal.*, *50*, 147, 1953.

Brini, A. and Payeur, G. — La kératite ponctuée superficielle de Thygeson (rappel clinique et thérapeutique à propos de deux cas). *Bull. Soc. Ophthal. Fr.*, *66*, 1282, 1966.

Briones, O.C., Hanna, L., Jawetz, E. et al. — Type-specific antibodies in human chlamydial trachomatis infections of the eye. *J. Immunol.*, *113*, 1262, 1974.

Burns, R.P. and Potter, M.H. — Epidemic keratoconjunctivitis due to type 19. *Amer. J. Ophthal.*, *81*, 27, 1976.

Caldwell, G.G., Lindsey, N.J., Wulff, W., Donnelly, D.D. and Bohl, F.N. — Epidemic of adenovirus type 7 acute conjunctivitis in swimmers. *Amer. J. Epidem.*, *99*, 230, 1974.

Chiba, S., Umetsu, M., Yamanaka, T., Hori, S., Nakao, T. and Fukui, S. — An outbreak of epidemic keratoconjunctivitis due to adenovirus type 8 in a babies home. *Tohoku J. exp. Med.*, *119*, 159, 1976.

Cockburn, T.A., Rowe, W.P. and Huebner, R.J. — Relationship of the 1951 Greeley, Colorado outbreak of conjunctivitis and pharyngitis to type 3 APC virus infection. *Amer. J. Hyg.*, *63*, 250, 1956.

Davidson, S.I. — Epidemic keratoconjunctivitis—a report of an outbreak which resulted in ward cross-infection. *Brit. J. Ophthal.*, *48*, 573, 1964.

Dawson, C.R., Hanna, L., Wood, T.R. and Despain, R. — Adenovirus type 8 keratoconjunctivitis in the United States III. Epidemiologic, clinical and microbiologic features. *Amer. J. Ophthal.*, *69*, 473, 1970.

Dawson, C.R., Hanna, L. and Togni, B. — Adenovirus type 8 infection in the United States IV. Observations on the pathogenesis of lesions in severe eye disease. *Arch. Ophthal.*, *87*, 258, 1972.

Dawson, C.R. — Lids, conjunctiva and lacrimal apparatus. Eye infections with chlamydia. *Arch. Ophthal.*, *93*, 854, 1975.

Derrick, E.H. — Swimming bath conjunctivitis, with a report of three possible cases and a note on its epidemiology. *Med. J. Aust.*, *2*, 334, 1943.

Desmyter, J., de Jong, J.C., Slaterus, K.W. and Verlaeckt, H. — Keratoconjunctivitis caused by adenovirus type 19. *Br. Med. J.*, *2*, 406, 1974.

Dudgeon, J., Bhargava, S.K. and Ross, C.A. — Treatment of adenovirus infection of the eye with 5-iodo-2'-deoxyuridine. A double blind trial. *Brit. J. Ophthal.*, *53*, 530, 1969.

Duke-Elder, S.: System of ophthalmology. *Diseases of the outer eye*. Vol. 8, part 1, H. Kimpton, London, 1965.

Duke-Elder, S. and Leigh, A.G. — System of Ophthalmology, Vol. VIII, *Diseases of the outer eye*, Part 2; Henry Kimpton, London, 1965.

Ellison, E.D., Kaufman, H.E. and Little, J.M. — Comparison of methods for the laboratory diagnosis of ocular adenovirus type 3 infection. *Invest. Ophthal.*, *8*, 484, 1969.

Evans, A.S. — Acute respiratory disease in University of Wisconsin students. *New Engl. J. Med.*, *256*, 377, 1957.

Forster, R.K., Dawson, C.R. and Schachter, J. — Late follow-up of patients with neonatal inclusion conjunctivitis. *Amer. J. Ophthal.*, *69*, 497, 1970.

Fowle, A.M.C., Cockeram, A. and Ormsby, H.L. — Virus isolations from patients with keratoconjunctivitis. *Amer. J. Ophthal.*, *40*, 180, 1955.

Fowle, A.M., Simmons, V. and Ormsby, H.L. — Adenoviruses from Canadian cases of keratoconjunctivitis. *Amer. J. Ophthal.*, *43*, 32, 1957.

Freyler, H. and Sehorst, W. — Keratoconjunctivitis epidemica. Bericht über eine Klinikepidemie. *Klin. Mbl. Augenheilk.*, *166*, 69, 1975.

Freyler, H. and Sehorst, W. — Das Schicksal der Hornhautinfiltrate bei Keratoconjunctivitis epidemica. Eine verlaufsstudie über $2\frac{1}{2}$ Jahre. *Wien. Klin. Wschr.*, *11*, 341, 1976.

Fuchs, E. — Keratitis punctata superficialis. *Wien. Klin. Wschr.*, *2*, 837, 1889.

Germanis, M. and Jeansson, S. — Ocular illness in association with adenovirus type 3 infection. *Scand. J. Infect. Dis.*, *5*, 243, 1973.

Golden, B., Mc Kee, A.P. and Coppel, S.P. — Epidemic keratoconjunctivitis: a new approach. *Trans. Am. Acad. Ophthal. Otolaryng.*, *75*, 1216, 1971.

Gordon, F.B. and Quan, A.L. — Occurrence of glycogen in inclusions of the psittacosis-lymphogranuloma venereum-trachoma agents. *J. Infect. Dis.*, *115*, 186, 1965.

Grayson, M. — Oculogenital disease and related conditions. In: *Diseases of the cornea*. The C.V. Mosby Company, London, 1979.

Grayston, J.T., Yang, Y.F., Johnston, P.B. and Liang-She, K. — Epidemic keratoconjunctivitis on Taiwan. Etiological and clinical studies. *Am. J. Trop. Med. Hyg.*, *13*, 492, 1964.

Grist, N.R., Bell, E.J. and Gardner, C.A. — Epidemic keratoconjunctivitis. A continuing study. *Health Bull.*, *28*, 47, 1970.

Gutter, B. and Becker, Y.: Trachoma agent RNA synthesis. *J. Mol. Biol.*, *66*, 239, 1972.

Guyer, B., O'Day, D.M., Hierholzer, J.C. and Schaffner, W. — Epidemic keratoconjunctivitis. A community outbreak of mixed adenovirus type 8 and type 19 infection. *J. Infect. Dis.*, *132*, 142, 1975.

Halberstaedter, L. and von Prowazek, S. — Zur aetiologie des Trachomas. *Deutsch. Med. Wschr.*, *33*, 1285, 1907.

Hanna, L., Jawetz, E., Briones, O. et al.: Antibodies to TRIC agents in matched human tears and sera. *J. Immunol.*, *110*, 1464, 1973.

Hansman, D.: Inclusion conjunctivitis. *Med. J. Aust.*, *1*, 151, 1969.

Hart, J.C.D., Barnard, D.L., Clarke, S.K.R. and Marmion, V.J. — Epidemic keratoconjunctivitis. A virological and clinical study. *Trans. Ophthalmol. Soc. U.K.*, *92*, 795, 1972.

Havener, W.H. — Ocular pharmacology. The C.V. Mosby Company, St. Louis, 1978.

Hecht, S.D., Hanna, L., Sery, T.W. and Jawetz, E. — Treatment of epidemic keratoconjunctivitis with idoxuridine (IDU). *Arch. Ophthal.*, *73*, 49, 1965.

Hierholzer, J.C., Guyer, B., O'Day, D. and Schaffner, W. — Adenovirus type 19 keratoconjunctivitis. *New Engl. J. Med.*, *290*, 1436, 1974.

Hirota, M. — On the cytopathogenic agents isolated in vitro from epidemic keratoconjunctivitis. *Folia Ophthal. Jap.*, *8*, 84, 1957.

Hogan, M.J. and Crawford, J.W. — Epidemic keratoconjunctivitis. *Amer. J. Ophthal.*, *25*, 1059, 1942.

Hogan, M.J. — Keratoconjunctivitis, the clinical characteristics of the California epidemic 1941-42. *Amer. J. Ophthal.*, *43*, 41, 1957.

Huebner, R.J. and Rowe, W.P. — Adenoviruses as etiologic agents in conjunctivitis and keratoconjunctivitis. *Am. J. Ophthal.*, *43*, 20, 1957.

Imre, G., Korchmaros, I., Geck, P., Nasz, I. and Dan, P. — Antigenic specificity of inclusion bodies in epidemic keratoconjunctivitis. *Ophthal.*, *148*, 7, 1964.

Inove, S. — Diagnosis of adenovirus infection by use of fluorescent antibody technique. *Acta Soc. Ophthal. Jap.*, *72*, 728, 1968.

Inove, S.A. — A study of epidemic keratoconjunctivitis. The use of fluorescent antibody techniques. *Acta Soc. Ophthal. Jap.*, *75*, 2180, 1971.

Ishizu, M. — The application of fluorescent antibody technique to studies of epidemic keratoconjunctivitis. *Acta Soc. Ophthal. Jap.*, *73*, 23, 1969.

Jackson, W.B., Davis, P.L., Groh, V. and Champlin, R. — Adenovirus type 19 keratoconjunctivitis in Canada. *Canad. J. Ophthal.*, *10*, 326, 1975.

Jansco, A. and Simons, M. — Aetiology of keratoconjunctivitis in epidemic and non epidemic periods. *Acta Microbiol. Acad. Sci. Hung.*, *12*, 123, 1965.

Jawetz, E., Kimura, S.J., Hanna, L., Coleman, V.R., Thygeson, P. and Nicholas, A. — Studies on the etiology of epidemic keratoconjunctivitis. *Amer. J. Ophthal.*, *40*, 200 (part 2), 1955.

Jawetz, E., Thygeson, P., Hanna, L., Nichols, A. and Kimura, S.J. — The etiology of epidemic keratoconjunctivitis. *Amer. J. Ophthal.*, *43*, 79, 1957.

Jones, B.R. — The differential diagnosis of punctate keratitis. *Trans. Ophthal. Soc. U.K.*, *80*, 665, 1960.

Jones, B.R. — Adenovirus infections of the eye in London. *Trans. Ophthal. Soc. U.K.*, *82*, 621, 1962.

Jones, B.R. — Thygeson's superficial punctate keratitis. *Trans. Ophthal. Soc. U.K.*, *83*, 245, 1963.

Jones, B.R., Darougar, S., Mohsenine, H. and Proirier, R.H. — Communicable ophthalmia: the blinding scourge of the Middle East. *Brit. J. Ophthal.*, *60*, 492, 1976.

Kasova, V. and Bruckova, M. — A mixed outbreak of epidemic keratoconjunctivitis due to adenovirus types 29 and 8. *Zbl. Bakt. Hyg.*, *239*, 1, 1977.

Kasova, V., Bruckova, M., Kotelensky, F., Kotelenska, K. and Ulrichova, R. — Isolation of adenovirus type 29 form an outbreak of epidemic keratoconjunctivitis. *Acta Virol.*, *21*, 173, 1977.

Kendall, E.J.C., Riddle, R.W., Tuck, H.A., Rodan, K.S., Andrews, B.E. and McDonald, J.C.: Pharyngo-conjunctival fever: school outbreak in England during the summer of 1955 associated with adenovirus types 3, 7, 14. *Brit. Med. J.*, *2*, 131, 1957.

Kimura, S.J., Hanna, L., Nichols, A., Thygeson, D. and Jawetz, E. — Sporadic cases of pharyngoconjunctival fever in Northern California. *Amer. J. Ophthal.*, *43*, 14, 1957.

Knopf, H.L.S. and Hierholzer, J.C. — Clinical and immunological responses in patients with viral keratoconjunctivitis. *Amer. J. Ophthal.*, *80*, 661, 1975.

Koseki, S. — Studies on adenovirus type 11 infection of the eye. *Jap. J. Ophthal.*, *4*, 92, 1960.

Laibson, P.R., Ortolan, G. and Dupre-Strachan, S. — Community and hospital outbreaks of epidemic keratoconjunctivitis. *Arch. Ophthal.*, *80*, 467, 1968.

Laibson, P.R. and Green, W.R. — Conjunctival membranes in epidemic keratoconjunctivitis. *Arch. Ophthal.*, *83*, 100, 1970.

Laibson, P.R., Dhiri, S., O'Conner, J. and Ortolan, G. — Corneal infiltrates in epidemic keratoconjunctivitis. *Arch. Ophthal.*, *84*, 36, 1970.

Laibson, P.R. — Adenoviral keratoconjunctivitis. *Int. Ophthal. Clinics*, *15*, 187, 1975.

Lemp, M.A., Chambers, R.W. and Lundy, J.: Viral isolate in superficial punctate keratitis. *Arch. Ophthal.*, *91*, 8, 1974.

Leopold, I.H. — Characteristics of hospital epidemics of epidemic keratoconjunctivitis. *Amer. J. Ophthal.*, *43*, 93, 1957.

Locatcher-Khorazo, D. and Seegal, B.C. — Microbiology of the eye. The C.V. Mosby Company, St. Louis, 1972.

Marre, M., Rhode, W. and Klier, G. — Isolierung und differenzierung von adenovirus typ 8 bei epidemischer keratoconjunctivitis in Liepzig. *Alb. v. Graefes Arch. Ophthal.*, *172*, 355, 1967.

McComb, D. E. and Nichols, R. L. — Antibody type specificity to trachoma in eye secretions of Saudi Arab children. *Infect. Immun.*, *2*, 65, 1970.

Mitsui, Y. and Suzuki, A. — Electron microscopy of trachoma virus in section. *Arch. Ophthal.*, *56*, 429, 1956.

Mitsui, Y., Hanabusa, J., Minoda, R. and Ogata, S. — Effect of inoculating adenovirus (APC) virus type 8 into human volunteers. *Amer. J. Ophthal.*, *43*, 84, 1957.

Mitsui, Y., Hanna, L., Hanabusa, J., Minoda, R., Ogata, S., Kurihara, H., Okamura, R. and Miura, M. — Association of adenovirus type 8 with epidemic keratoconjunctivitis. *Arch. Ophthal.*, *61*, 891, 1959.

Muzzi, A., Rocchi, G., Lumbroso, B., Tosato, G. and Barberi, F. — Acute haemorrhagic conjunctivitis during an epidemic outbreak of adenovirus type 4 infection. *Lancet*, *2*, 822, 1975.

O'Day, D. M., Guyer, B., Hiermolzer, J. C., Rosing, K. J. and Schaffner, W. — Clinical and laboratory evaluation of epidemic keratoconjunctivitis due to adenovirus types 8 and 19. *Amer. J. Ophthal.*, *81*, 207, 1976.

Okamura, R. — A study of pharyngoconjunctival fever. *Acta Soc. Ophthal. Jap.*, *64*, 96, 1960.

Oker-Blom, N., Wager, O., Strandström, H., Makela, P., and Jansson, E. — Adenovirus associated with pharyngoconjunctival fever. *Ann. Med. Exp. Biol. Fenn.*, *35*, 342, 1957.

Ormsby, H. L. and Aitchison, W. S. — The role of the swimming pool in the transmission of pharyngoconjunctival fever. *Canad. Med. Ass. J.*, *73*, 864, 1955.

Ormsby, H. L., Fowle, A. M. L. and Doane, F. — Canadian cases of adenovirus infection 1951-56. *Amer. J. Ophthal.*, 43, 17, 1957.

Ostler, H. B. — Oculogenital disease. *Surv. Ophthal.*, *20*, 223, 1976.

Pavan.Langston, D. and Dohlman, C. H. — A double blind clinical study of adenine arabinoside therapy of viral keratoconjunctivitis. *Amer. J. Ophthal.*, *74*, 81, 1972.

Perkins, H. R. and Allison, A. C. — Cell-wall constituents of rickettsiae and psittacosis-lymphogranuloma organisms. *J. Gen. Microbiol.*, *30*, 469, 1963.

Pirouz, M. S. — Trois cas de kératite ponctuée superficielle de Thygeson. *Ann. Oculist.*, *210*, 509, 1977.

Profeta, M. L., Verdi, G. P. and Orzalesi, N. — Epidemia di cheratoconjunctivite epidemica (CCE) da adenovirus tipo 9. *Ann. Sclavo*, 1963.

Quere, M. A., Diallo, J. and Rogez, J. P. — La kératite de Thygeson (a propos de 16 cas de kératite ponctuée superficielle). *Bull. Soc. Ophthal. Fr.*, *67*, 276, 1967.

Quere, M. A., Diallo, J. and Rogez, J. P. — La kératite de Thygeson. *Arch. Ophtal.*, *28*, 497, 1968.

Quere, M. A., Delplace, M. P., Rossazza, C., Moulene, C. and Combe, J. — Fréquence et étiopathogénie de la kératite de Thygeson. *Bull. Soc. Ophtal. Fr.*, *73*, 535, 1973.

Reid, D., Bell, E. J., Grist, N. R., Taylor, J. C. and Ellis, J. R. — Epidemic keratoconjunctivitis in the West of Scotland. 1967-72. *J. Hyg. (Camb.)*, *73*, 157, 1974.

Rowe, W. P., Huebner, R. J., Gilmor, L. K., Parrott, R. H. and Ward, T. G. — Isolation of cytopathogenic agent from human adenoids undergoing spontaneous degeneration in tissue culture. *Proc. Soc. Exp. Biol. Med.*, *84*, 570, 1953.

Rowe, W. P., Huebner, R. J., Hartley, J. W., Ward, T. G. and Parrott, R. H. — Studies of the adenoidal-pharyngeal conjunctival (APC) group of viruses. *Amer. J. Hyg.*, *61*, 197, 1955.

Sarov, I. and Becker, Y. — Trachoma agent DNA. *J. Mol. Biol.*, *42*, 581, 1963.

Sarov, I. and Becker, Y. — RNA in the elementary bodies of trachoma agent. *Nature*, *217*, 849, 1968.

Sarov, I. and Becker, Y. — DNA dependent RNA polymerase in trachoma elementary bodies. In: *Trachoma and related disorders caused by chlamydial agents*. Nichols, R. L. Ed. Excerpta Medica, Amsterdam, 1971 a.

Sarov, I. and Becker, Y. — DNA-dependent RNA polymerase in purified trachoma elementary bodies: effect of Nall on RNA transcription. *J. Bacteriol.*, *107*, 593, 1971 b.

Segawa, K. — Epidemic keratoconjunctivitis: light and electron microscopic study on the conjunctival epithelium. *Jap. J. Ophthal.*, *6* (pt. 3), 143, 1962.
Silverstein, A.M. — The immunologic modulation of infections disease pathogenesis. *Invest. Ophthal.*, *13*, 560, 1974.
Sugiura, S., Koike, K., Yokoyama, Y. and Kondo, Y. — The role of adenovirus type 3 and type 7 infection in epidemic keratoconjunctivitis (EKC). *Acta Soc. Ophthal. Jap.*, *63*, 3452, 1959.
Sundmacher, R., Neumann-Haefelin, D. and Bettge, F. — Kératitis superficialis punctate Thygeson. Tagung der Berliner Augenärztlichen Gesellschaft 1975. *Klin. Monatsbl. Augenheilk.*, *168*, 868, 1976.
Sundmacher, R., Press, M., Neumann- Haefelin, D. and Riede, U. — Keratitis superficialis punctata Thygeson. *Klin. Monatsbl. Augenheilk.*, *170*, 908, 1977.
Tang, F., Chang, H., Huang, Y. and Wang, K. — Studies of the etiology of trachoma with special reference to isolation of the virus in chick embryo. *Chin. Med. J.*, *75*, 429, 1957.
Tanifuji, Y., Mita, K., Sato, Y., Isikava, Y., Sase, Y. and Kondo, T. — Outbreak of acute conjunctivitis caused by adenovirus type 3. *Folia Ophthal. Jap.*, *25*, 1, 1974.
Thygeson, P., Proctor, F.I. and Richards, P. — Etiologic significance of the elementary body in trachoma. *Amer. J. Ophthal.*, *18*, 811, 1935.
Thygeson, P. — Superficial punctate keratitis. *J.A.M.A.*, *144*, 1544, 1950.
Thygeson, P. — Office and dispensary transmissions of epidemic keratoconjunctivitis. *Amer. J. Ophthal.*, *43*, 98, 1957.
Thygeson, P. — Further observations on superficial punctate keratitis. *Arch. Ophthal.*, *66*, 158, 1961.
Thygeson, P. — Clinical and laboratory investigations on superficial punctate keratitis. *Amer. J. Ophthal.*, *61*, 1344, 1966.
Thygeson, P. — Historical review of oculogenital disease. *Amer. J. Ophthal.*, *71*, 975, 1971.
Tommila, V. and Lapinleimu, K. — A hospital epidemic of keratoconjunctivitis caused by adenovirus type 7 in Helsinki. *Acta Ophthal. (kbh)*, *43*, 294, 1965.
Tullo, A.B. and Higgins, P.G. — Epidemic adenovirus keratoconjunctivitis. *Lancet*, 442, 1978.
Uchida, Y.V. and Inove, S. — Fluorescent antibody studies of epidemic keratoconjunctivitis. *Tokushima J. Exp. Med.*, *14*, 13, 1967.
Van der Veen, J. and Van der Ploeg — An outbreak of pharyngo-conjunctival fever caused by types 3 and 4 adenovirus at Waalrijk, The Netherlands. *Amer. J. Hyg.*, *68*, 95, 1958.
Vastine, D.W., West, C.E., Yamashiroya, H., Smith, R., Saxtan, D.C., Gieser, D.I. and Mufson, M.A. — Simultaneous nosocomial and community outbreak of epidemic keratoconjunctivitis with types 8 and 19 adenovirus. *Trans. Amer. Acad. Ophthal. Otolaryng.*, *81*, op 826, 1976.
Vastine, D.W., Schwartz, H.S., Yamashiroya, H.M., Smith, R.F. and Guth, S.B. — Cytologic diagnosis of adenoviral epidemic keratoconjunctivitis by direct immunofluorescence. *Invest. Ophthal. and Vis. Sci.*, *16*, 195, 1977.
Vorgosko, A.J., Kim, H.W., Parrott, R.H., Jefferies, B.C., Wong, D. and Chanock, R.M. — Recovery and identification of adenovirus in infections of infants and children. *Bacteriological Reviews*, *29*, 487, 1965.
Wang, S.P., Kuo, C.C. and Grayston, J.T. — A simplified method for immunological typing of trachoma-inclusion conjunctivitis-lymphogranuloma venereum organisms. *Infect. Immuno.*, *7*, 356, 1973.
Wang, S.P. and Grayston, J.T. — Human serology in chlamydia trachomatis infection with microimmunofluorescence. *J. Infect. Dis.*, *130*, 388, 1974.
Ward, T.G., Huebner, R.J., Rowe, W.P., Ryan, R.W. and Bell, J.A. — Production of pharyngoconjunctival fever in human volunteers inoculated with APC viruses. *Science*, *122*, 1086, 1955.
Warring III, G.O., Laibson, P.R., Satz, J.E. and Joseph, N.H. — Use of vidarabine in epidemic keratoconjunctivitis due to adenovirus types 3, 7, 8 and 19. *Amer. J. Ophthal.*, *82*, 781, 1976.

Wassileva, P.I. and Galabov, A.S. — Über die Behandlung der epidemischen Kerato-conjunctivitis mit ABOB. *Klin. Mbl. Augenheil.*, *166*, 77, 1975.
W.H.O. — Expert Committee on Trachoma. *Tech. Report*, Ser. No. 234, 1962.
Wigand, R., Bruch, P. and Keckenhan, K. — Untersuchungen zur ätiologie der epidemischen Keratoconjunktivitis. *Klin. Mbl. Augenheilk.*, *167*, 823, 1975.
Yoneda, C., Dawson, C.R., Daghfous, T., Hoshiwara, I., Jones, P., Messadi, M. and Schachter, J. — Cytology as a guide to the presence of chlamydial inclusions in Giemsa-stained conjunctival smears in severe endemic trachoma. *Brit. J. Ophthal.*, *59*, 116, 1975.
Zografos, L. — La kérato-conjunctivite de l'adeno-virus type 10. *Ophtal.*, *174*, 61, 1977.
Zweighaft, R.M., Hierholzer, J.C. and Bryan, J.A. — Epidemic keratoconjunctivitis at a Vietnamese refugee camp in Florida. *Amer. J. Epidem.*, *106*, 399, 1977.

CHAPTER VIII

THE HERPES VIRUS

The word "herpes" (to creep) has been used in medicine since ancient times to describe a variety of skin conditions until the ninteenth century. The material excreted from the lesions was thaught to be bile mixed with other humors (Wildy, 1973). Since the fourth decade of this century, rapid developments in the understanding of viral diseases have considerably changed the concept of herpesvirus infections.

To date, more than 60 herpesviruses are known to infect over 30 different birds, animals and man (Watson, 1973; Lennartz, 1979). The herpesvirus particle measures 100-150 nm, containing a double stranded DNA core, surrounded by an icosahedral capsid with 162 hollow capsomeres (fig. VIII-1) with a lipid containing membrane which makes it sensitive to lipid solvents like ether. Development of the virus begins in the nucleus and is completed by acquiring an outer envelope derived from the host cell membranes as the virus passes into the cytoplasm.

At least four morphologically indistinguishable members of this large virus group are known to cause disease in man: herpes simplex, herpes zoster (Varicella-Zoster), Epstein-Barr (EB) virus (infectious mononucleosis), and human cytomegalovirus.

HERPES SIMPLEX

Epidemiology

Herpes simplex virus (HSV) infections are one of the most common viral diseases of man with world-wide distribution. Vidal (1873), first showed the infectious nature of herpes simplex by human inoculation experiments and Grüter in 1912 successfully transferred herpetic keratitis from man to rabbit eyes (Grüter, 1920 a and b).

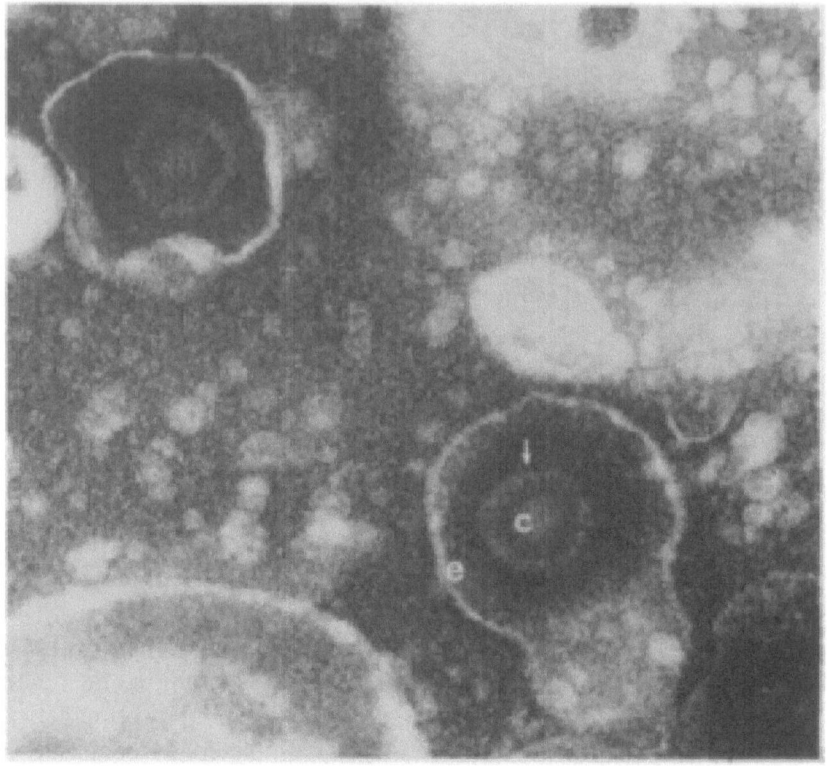

Fig. VIII-1. — Herpesvirus particles in a phosphotungstic acid negative stained preparation. The central DNA core (c) is surrounded by a capsid (arrow). The outer envelope (e) is derived from the host-cell membrane. (Courtesy of Prof. J. Desmeyter and Dr. G. De Groote).

The primary infection occurs usually before 5 years of age. In USA 60% of the population showed antiherpes serum neutralizing antibodies by 5 years age which increased to 90% by 15 years age (Buddingh et al., 1953). At 60 years age 97% of the population may show serum antibodies (Smith et al., 1967). In low socio-economic groups living in poor hygienic conditions the incidence of HSV infections may vary from 90-100% and in higher socio-economic groups living in good hygienic conditions it is only 50-60% (Buddingh et al., 1953; MacCallum, 1959; Duke-Elder, 1965). Over 60% of infected persons may be the life long carriers of the virus (Germer, 1954). Herpes virus has been isolated from saliva and stools of 5-7% of healthy individuals of all ages (Nasemann, 1979).

In general, infants are protected by maternal antibodies upto 6 months after birth but this protection is not absolute. A primary infection may occur due to contamination from mother's genital tract during delivery. Such infections are usually systemic and may be fatal. Neonatal infections may present with keratoconjunctivitis, gingivostomatitis, eczema herpeticum, meningo-encephalitis with or without visceral involvement, i.e.; lungs, adrenal cortex, kidney, liver, spleen, bone-marrow infections (Haas, 1935; Quilligan and Wilson, 1951; Zuelzar and Stulberg, 1952; France and Wilmers, 1953). Herpetic encephalitis (primary or secondary) may lead to death in adults (Zorafonetis et al., 1944; Whitman et al., 1946). According to Söltz-Szötz (1959) two types of antibodies develop after herpes virus infection. Virus-bound, "V-antibodies (IgM)", remain at a constant titer after primary infection while the soluble-antibodies, "S-antibodies (IgG)", decrease before each clinical recurrence.

Two types of herpes simplex viruses are recognized to produce disease in human beings. HSV type 1, generally causes infections of the upper respiratory tract, gingivo stomatitis, eye and cutancous infections. HSV type 2, is responsible for ano-genital and neonatal infections. Both types of the viruses, however, may affect all areas of the body. Also, type 2 virus is thought to be related to cervical cancer in females.

Primary infections

Primary HSV infection usually occurs early in life, i.e. before 5 years of age, but may occur at any age. The incubation period varies from 2 to 12 days. According to Leopold and Serry (1963) and Locatcher-Khorazo and Seegal (1972), the infection remains subclinical in 85-90% of cases. Wheeler (1972), on the other hand, believes that some degree of clinical disease appears in about half of the patients. Usually the symptoms are few and minimal. Recovery takes place in a few days to a few weeks even if the symptoms are severe. Occasionally severe illness may be fatal (Ostler, 1976 a).

Ocular lesions

Primary infection

Primary HSV infection may involve the lids or skin around the eyes. It is typically unilateral (fig. VIII-2) but may be bilateral.

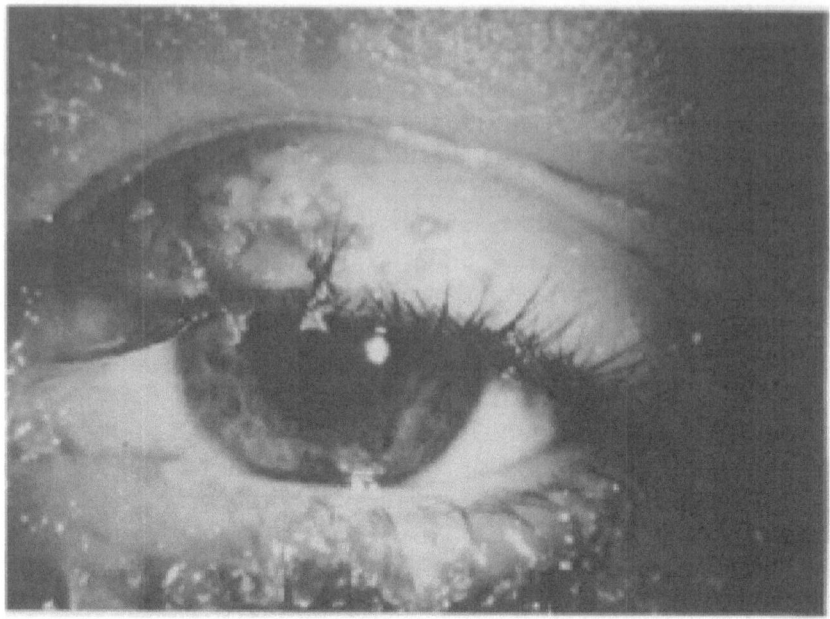

Fig. VIII-2. — Herpes simplex virus infection of the eyelids.

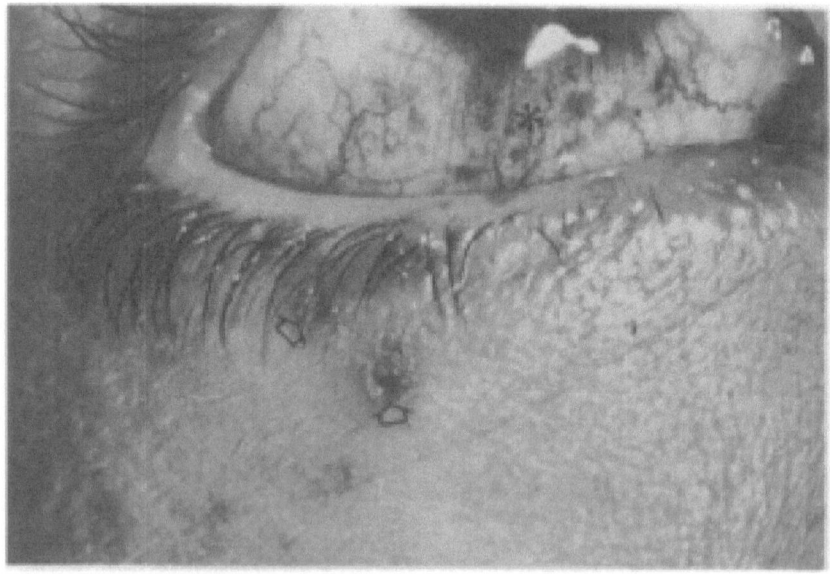

Fig. VIII-3. — Skin lesions (arrows), and conjunctivitis marked by ecchymoses (*). Herpes simplex virus infection.

Vesicles appear on one or both eyelid margins with edema and pain. Other areas of the face may be involved (Gunderson, 1936). Main feature of the primary eye infection is follicular conjunctivitis which may precede keratitis or other lesions by several days. According to some authors eye symptoms are quite common in primary HSV infection, but their herpetic origin would usually not be recognised. Sometimes, subconjunctival ecchymoses (fig. VIII-3), conjunctival pseudo-membranes, or conjunctival dendritic lesions develop (Laibson, 1973). In about two third of the cases corneal involvement occurs in the form of fine or coarse epithelial lesions. Dendritic, geographical or metaherpetic ulcers may develop in exceptional cases. Corneal filaments and vesicular keratitis has also been reported in primary infections (Thygeson, 1959). There is associated pain, photophobia, lacrimation and some mucoid discharge. As the characteristic corneal hypoesthesia develops the symptoms of pain and blepharospasm become less severe. Medium sized white keratic precipitates may appear on the posterior cornea just behind the epithelial lesions. There may be minimal aqueous flare with iritis and cellular infiltration of the iris. The iritis is thought to be reactive type mediated by the prostaglandines. According to Ostler (1976a), severe iritis is exceptional in primary HSV infections of the newborn but regional lymphadenopathy is the rule. In most instances the primary HSV eye infection would heal without scar formation.

Primary herpes simplex infections may be very severe in atopic patients (Easty et al., 1975; Dawson and Togni, 1976).

Herpes simplex eye lesions have been described to be present at birth (Hagler et al., 1969; Pettay et al., 1972; Hutchison et al., 1975) or may develop in the neonatal period (Batignani, 1934; Smith et al., 1941; Pillard et al., 1950; Zuelzer and Stulberg, 1952; Florman and Mindlin, 1952; Monnet et al., 1961; Neimann et al., 1963; Langvad and Voigt, 1963; Mitchell and McCall, 1963; Cogan et al., 1964; Yen et al., 1965; Bahrani et al., 1966; Berkovich and Ressel, 1966; Proto and Tedesco, 1966; May et al., 1967; Partridge and Millis, 1968; Golden et al., 1969; Hagler et al., 1969; Bobo et al., 1970; Nahmias et al., 1970; Cibis and Burde, 1971; Nahmias et al., 1976). About half of these infants were born premature and showed involvement of central nervous system, skin, cornea, conjunctiva, viscera, eyelids, oral cavity and optic neuritis, choreoretinitis, cataracts and microphthalmia in various combinations and severity. Conjunctivitis may precede any other signs of clinical disease. About 80% of the infections are caused by HSV type 2.

Infection is believed to occur during passage through mother's infected genital tract during delivery or an ascending infection through premature rupture of membranes. However, in the case of Hutchison et al. (1975) the mother had no evidence of genital herpes, the cervical cultures for virus isolation were negative and the twins were delivered by caesarean section without prior rupture of membranes. Only one of the twins at birth showed HSV type 1 uniocular infection with skin lesions, conjunctivitis and geographic corneal ulcer. Since the keratitis was quite advanced, the infection could have occurred in utero only through placenta or an ascending infection through intact membranes. This case demonstrates that in utero infections may be responsible for some of the congenital ocular anomalies.

Latent infection

After a primary infection the virus enters a stage of symbiosis and may be shed from time to time in tears, saliva, respiratory secretions and stools without producing clinical disease (Lindgren et al., 1968). However, in some patients it may be responsible for recurrences over prolonged periods or whole life. Originally the lacrimal gland was thought to be the site of latent infection (Kaufman et al., 1968) as virus could be cultured from tears before recurrence of keratitis (Kaufman et al., 1967; Nesburn et al., 1967; Brown et al., 1968; Laibson et al., 1969). Since the virus could be isolated from the rabbit orbital cavity after enucleation (Brown and Kaufman, 1969), the cornea was excluded as the site of latent infection. Pavan-Langston and Nesburn (1968) on the other hand, recovered HSV only once out of 96 lacrimal glands of rabbit. The theory of lacrimal gland involvement persisted till the virus was demonstrated in sensory ganglia.

Following the experimental studies of herpetic keratitis by Löwenstein (1919) and Grüter (1920 a and b) neurological involvement of some rabbits with herpetic eye disease was noted (Doerr, 1920; Doerr and Vöchting, 1920). Further experiments lead to the belief that the virus spreads to the nervous system from the periphery through axons (Goodpasture and Teague, 1923; and Goodpasture, 1925 a and b).

On the basis of these experiments and clinical observations, Good-pasture (1929) suggested the possibility of a latent viral infection of the neural ganglia. The early experiments of neuronal involvement have been recently confirmed (Wildy, 1967; Cook and Stevens, 1974). The experimental proof of this theory, however, came only in 1971, when Stevens and Cook isolated herpes simplex virus from the spinal ganglia of mice many months after herpes simplex infection.

Soon, thereafter, Nesburn et al. (1972); and Knotts et al. (1973) demonstrated the latent virus in trigeminal ganglion of rabbits, while it was not detected in any of the ocular adnexa, cornea, iris or trigeminal nerve of rabbits or mice. Knotts et al. (1973) also detected latent virus in the fifth nerve nucleus of some of the animals. Bastian et al. (1972) and Baringer and Swoveland (1973) recovered HSV from human trigeminal ganglia and Baringer (1974) from human sacral ganglia. The observation that the virus can only be recovered in organ culture shows that it is a latent infection.

Transplant studies provide additonial support for the neuronal theory (Kibrik and Gooding, 1965). When skin from an area of recurrent herpes is transplanted elsewhere in the body; it does not develop herpetic lesions but healthy skin transplanted to the site of recurrent infections may develop new lesions.

In a recent study (Mintsioulis et al., 1979), iritis, conjunctivitis and in some animals dendritic keratitis developed after inoculation of HSV in the superior cervical ganglion of rabbit. Virus isolations were done from uveal-retinal preparations and conjunctival swabbings. Other sensory ganglia of mouse, rabbit and guinae pig may harbour latent virus after inoculation with HSV on different body areas (Stevens et al., 1972; Knotts et al., 1973; Walz et al., 1974; Scriba, 1975).

It has been suggested that the latent virus is maintained in neurons in nonreplicating stage due to the modulating influence of specific immune IgG (Cook and Stevens, 1974, Stevens and Cook, 1974). However, this opinion is challanged by the observation that serum antibody levels are unrelated to the clinical recurrences (Chang, 1971). Also the serum antibody levels are unrelated to antibodies in saliva or oral infections (Douglas and Couch, 1970). Similarly the ocular recurrences are not related to the secretary antibodies in tears (Locatcher-Khorazo and Seegal, 1972). The biological process leading to the stimulation of virus growth and spreading is not understood.

Recurrent infection

The recurrence of herpetic disease in spite of the presence of circulating specific antibodies may be a secondary infection or the reactivation of latent virus. Repeated episodes of disease in recurrent infection tend to manifest on the same site but may involve other areas than the primary infection.

The biochemical basis for latency and reactivation is unknown. Surgical resection of the trigeminal root for the treatment of tic douloureux may lead to the reactivation of herpes lesions (Carton and Kilbourne, 1952). However, if the virus is not localized in the ganglion cells of any of the trigeminal nerve divisions, the herpetic disease does not appear in the segment supplied by that particular division (Baringer, 1976). In experimental animals retrobulbar disruption of trigeminal nerve function or the stereotaxic interruption of intracranial trigeminal nerve function prior to primary HSV infection, leads to marked decrease in virus isolations from the eye or recurrent disease. On the other hand stereotaxic or neurosurgical stimulation of the trigeminal ganglion in chronically infected animals produces a significant increase in virus isolation (Nesburn et al., 1976a and b). These experiments also demonstrate that the latent HSV from the trigeminal ganglion is transmitted to the ocular tissues through the trigeminal nerve.

The mechanism of reflex trigeminal ganglion stimulation may be operative in patients developing corneal herpes after foreign bodies or corneal injuries. Ocular episodes may appear as response to other stimuli or "triggers"; the most common of which are fever, exposure to sunlight or ultraviolet light, cold wind, overwork, psychological disturbances and menstruation (Dawson and Togni, 1976; Binder, 1977).

Reactivation of virus or keratitis in rabbits can be produced on epinephrine administration, many months after the recovery from primary infection (Laibson and Kibrick, 1966 and 1967). Tokumaru (1971) showed that capillary dilatation and hemorrhagic spots develop in rabbits if epinephrine is injected in skin 3 to 4 hours after inoculation of HSV at the same site. It is suggested that a similar vascular effect may be produced at the site of latent infection on systemic epinephrine administration which might play a role in viral reactivation. Recurrent HSV infections may cause blepharitis, blepharocojunctivitis or acute follicular conjunctivitis alone (Dawson and Togni, 1976).

Recurrent conjunctival ulceration is rare (Nauheim, 1969).

Recurrent punctate keratitis

Although the most frequent corneal lesion of recurrent HSV corneal infection is a branching linear "dendritic ulcer", sometimes coarse punctate (fig. VIII-4), areolar (comma shaped), or stellate (star shaped or microdendritic) lesions may develop on the cornea (Dawson and Togni, 1976; Maudgal and Missotten, 1979b). The attack begins with pain, irritation and lacrimation with some reduction in vision and photophobia. Usually the eye becomes red but occasionally in some patients may remain conspicuously white. With slit lamp biomicroscopy, initially, fine granular epithelial spots associated with epithelial bedewing and occasionally transient delicate vesicles may be seen (Duke-Elder, 1965). The rupture of vesicles causes

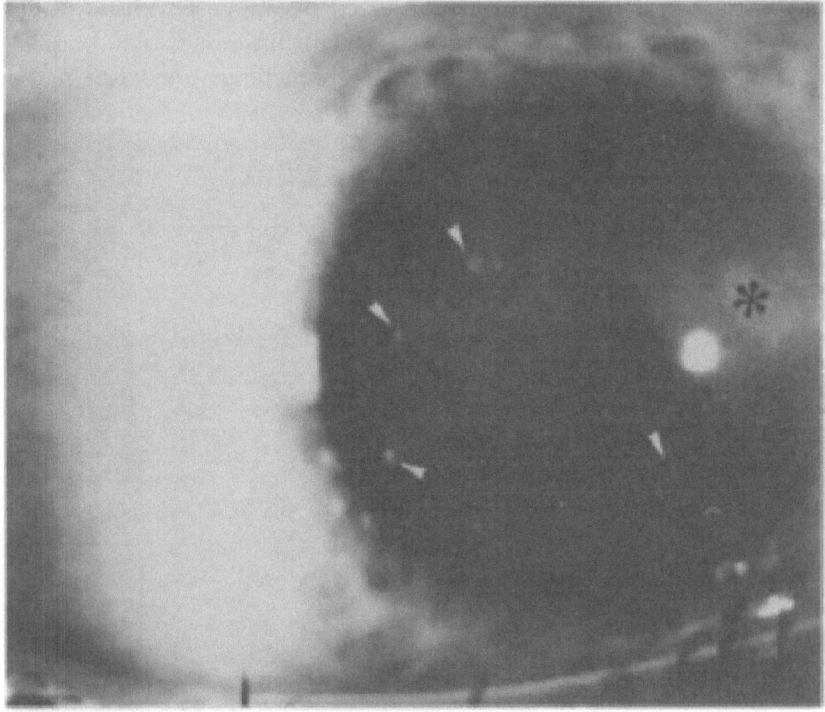

Fig. VIII-4. — Herpes simplex punctate keratitis (arrows). To the right a diffuse scar (*) of old keratitis is present.

intense pain. Fusion of punctate spots may result in variable shaped coarse punctate, areolar, stellate or microdendritic lesions. There is palisading of surrounding epithelial cells around the lesions (Binder, 1977), a sign of considerable diagnostic importance in our experience. Fluorescein stains all the lesions and in a few minutes may infiltrate into a considerable area around the lesion where epithelium is loosely attached to Bowman's membrane. Greyish stromal infiltrates may develop rapidly posterior to the epithelial lesions. The keratitis may heal in a few days to a few weeks without scarring. However, coalescence of punctate spots may lead to dendrite formation (Binder, 1977).

Dendritic ulcers

These ulcers may develop in any location on the cornea, irrespective of the site of primary lesions. After a first attack the recurrence rate varies from 18 to 25% (Laibson and Leopold, 1964; Hughes, 1969; De Voe, 1972; Binder, 1977) but after two or mare attacks may rise to 43% in two years (Carroll et al., 1967). Dendritic ulcers show linear irregular shape (fig. VIII-5) with numerous side branchings with terminal nodes at the end of branchings and also in the

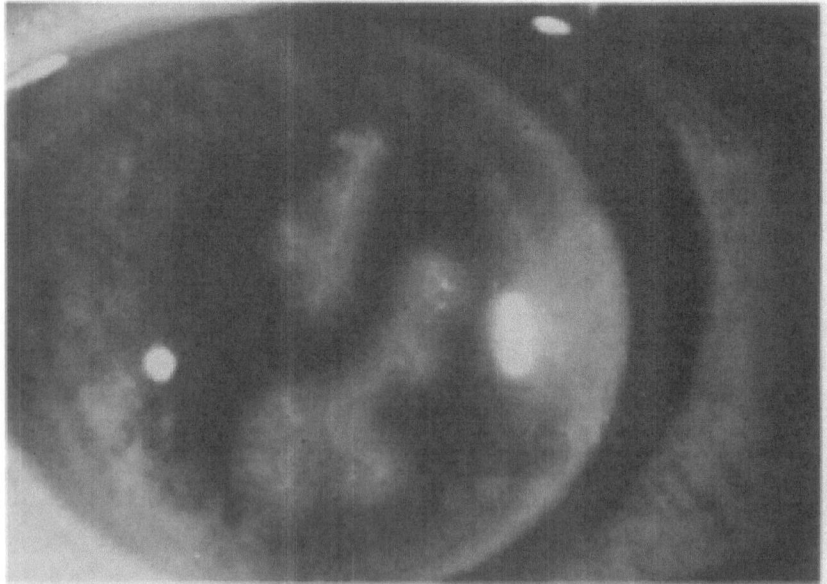

Fig. VIII-5. — Typical herpes simplex virus dendritic ulcers of the cornea. Fluorescein staining.

body of the lesions, especially where the side branches originate. Like in punctate lesions there is palisading of epithelium along the dendritic figure which contains large swollen cells of different sizes. The dendritic ulcer is stained by fluorescein, especially the slits between the swollen cells. Diffusion of fluorescein under the surrounding epithelium occurs like in punctate lesions. There may be slight stromal infiltration behind the dendritic ulcer. The dendritic ulcers may heal in a few weeks to some months without scar formation. Vascularization does not occur in epithelial disease. The ulcers persist longer and have increased tendency to recur in corneas with decreased sensitivity (Duke-Elder, 1965). Marginal dendritic ulcers as well as geographic or ameboid ulcers near the limbus take longer to heal, despite of antiviral therapy, than the central herpetic lesions (Sood and Marimon, 1964; Thygeson, 1971; Lanier, 1976) and tend to become chronic trophic ulcers (Pavan-Langston, 1975 a).

Geographic ulcers

Quite often, especially if corticosteroids are used, the dendritic ulcer broadens by necrosis of the swollen epithelial cells in the lesion. The resulting epithelial ulcer may assume a variety of geographic or amoeboid patterns (figs. VIII-6 and VIII-7). In uncomplicated cases we found that the stroma in the base of the ulcer may be remarkably clear or only minimally infiltrated but marked infiltration of stroma is the rule if corticosteroids have been used or secondary infection supervenes. There may be associated hypopyon and iridocyclitis (Duke-Elder, 1975).

HSV has been isolated less frequently from geographic ulcers than from dendritic lesions, but these ulcers take much longer to heal, often a few months (Hanna et al., 1957; Whitcher et al., 1976; Binder, 1977). In our experience the longer a geographic ulcer persists, the higher the risk of its becoming a persistent trophic ulcer. Healing takes place with some amount of corneal opacity, depending on the stromal involvement. Patients with iritis and hypopyon may have a poor prognosis (Duke-Elder, 1975).

Trophic corneal ulcers

After prolonged epithelial geographic ulceration or stromal herpetic involvement the surrounding epithelium may fail to grow over the epithelial defect (fig. VIII-8) even in the absence of active viral or

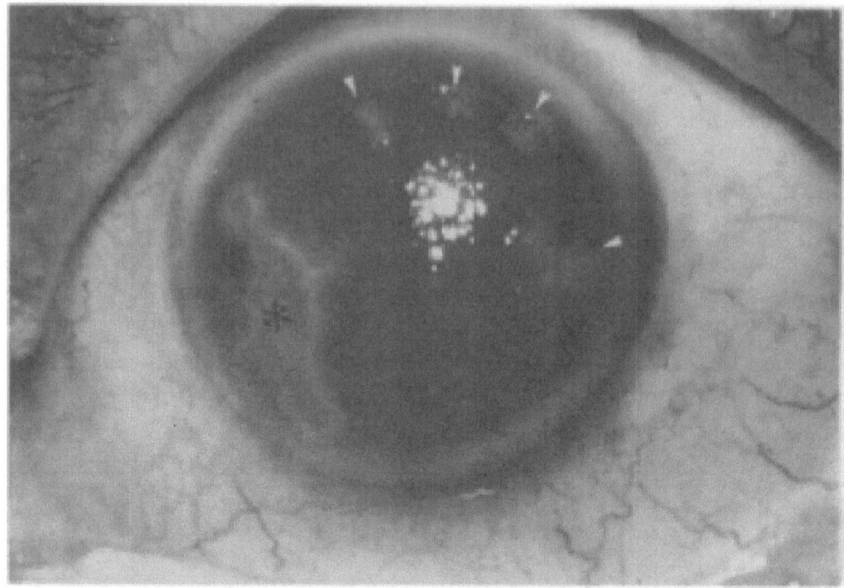

Fig. VIII-6. — Geographic ulcer (*) of the cornea with peripheral small ulcers (arrows) in herpes simplex keratitis.

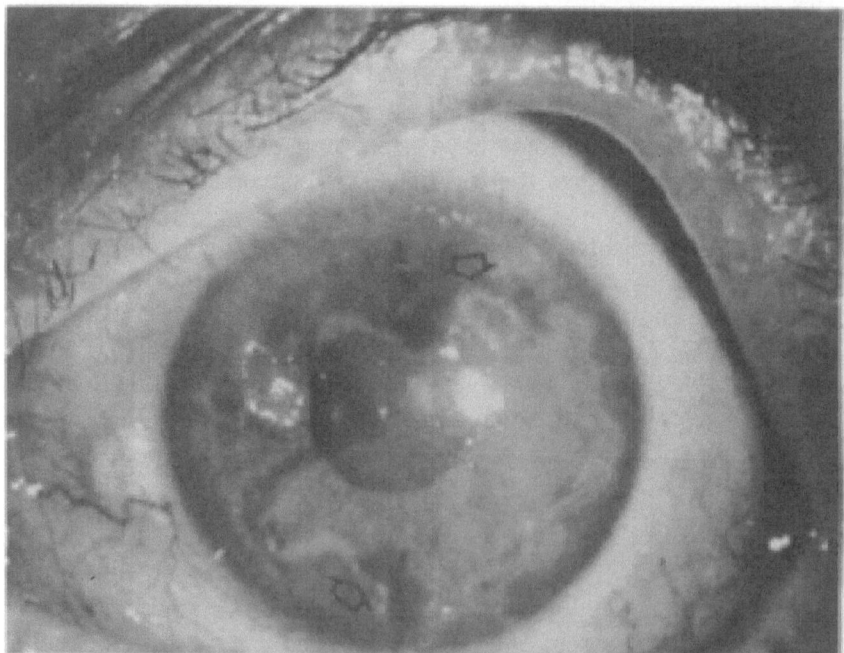

Fig. VIII-7. — Large amoeboid corneal ulcer caused by herpes simplex virus.

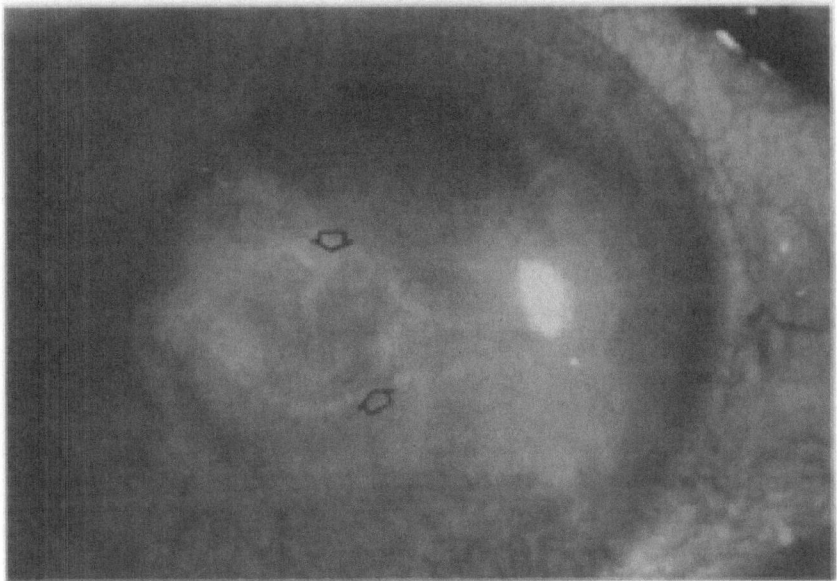

Fig. VIII-8. — Trophic corneal ulcer after herpes simplex keratitis. Arrows indicate the boundaries of the epithelium defect.

bacterial infection (Binder, 1977). If the epithelium grows over, it soon breaks down, probably due to a defective basement membrane and loosely attached epithelium. Loss of epithelium leads to corneal swelling and folds in Descemets' membrane. Since there is loss of sensitivity of the cornea they are termed as "trophic ulcers" or due to their resistence to treatment "indolent ulcers".

According to Kaufman (1964), the failure of regrowth of the corneal epithelium is due to the lack of epithelial basement membrane, like in recurrent erosions. Dohlman (1979), on the other hand, believes that the basic problem in these cases may be the mitotic arrest and inhibition of cell sliding at the edge of the epithelial defect related to the ratio of cyclic AMP and cyclic GMP content in the cells.

Stromal involvement

Every herpetic lesion of the cornea produces a slight opacification of the anterior stroma having the form of the dendritic lesions. These opacities are believed to be the product of antigen-antibody reaction as the viral antigens diffuse into stroma. These "ghost" or "phantom" lesions gradually disappear in many months (Dawson and Togni, 1976). Other stromal lesions in HSV infection may be disciform keratitis and focal or diffuse stromal keratitis.

Metaherpetic keratitis

In metaherpetic keratitis (Gundersen, 1936) there is associated stromal involvement with necrosis of collagen lamellae. It is believed that the stromal ulceration is produced by the increased collagenases and proteinases and other substances secreted by HSV infected epithelium (Itoi et al., 1969; Brown and Weller, 1970; Dohlman, 1979) or leucocytes attracted by the immune complexes in the stroma. Increased collagenolytic activity in rabbit corneas infected experimentally with HSV was shown by McCulley et al. (1970). Therefore, anticollagenase inhibitors may be of some benefit in the treatment of these ulcers. However, corneal melting and perforation may occur in spite of treatment.

Histopathology and Pathogenesis

Lipschütz (1921) described intranuclear inclusions in epithelial cells in herpetic skin lesions and later in herpetic keratitis. Cowdry (1934) classified A and B types of intranuclear inclusions. The type A inclusion is characterized by margination and condensation of nuclear chromatin on the nuclear membrane and a central intranuclear acidophillic mass separated from the marginated nuclear chromatin by a clear space or halo. Type B inclusions appear as masses in the nucleus. There is less nuclear degeneration, and margination of nuclear chromatin is absent. Thygeson (1958), studying the epithelial scrapings of dendritic corneal ulcers could not find intranuclear inclusions with certainty but reported the occurrence of multinucleated giant cells to be of diagnostic significance in HSV infection. Naib et al. (1967), however, stated that Cowdry type A inclusions are present only at an advanced stage of the disease. Nowakovsky et al. (1968) described intranuclear inclusions and syncytia formation in cervical scrapings of virologically positive HSV infection of genital tract in patients. Plotkin et al. (1971) described the development of Cowdry type A inclusions in the scraped corneal epithelium of HSV infected rabbit eyes. The inclusions could be detected one day post infection but were most numerous on 2nd and 3rd days. Similar inclusions have been described by Spinak (1978). Duke Elder (1965) summarized the histological findings of earlier authors who described the early hypertrophy of the nucleus, infoldings and thickening of the nuclear membrane; margination, aggregation or fragmentation of the nuclear chromatin; development of the large basophillic inclusion bodies and balloon degeneration of cells. These changes have been confirmed and further elaborated in comparative light and electron microscopic studies.

Scanning electron microscopy of experimental HSV keratitis shows the earliest epithelial lesions as small indented punctate areas involving 5 to 10 cells. The affected cells are depressed and arranged like the petals of a flower (Hollenberg et al., 1976). Transmission electron microscopy shows virus particles in the nuclei of the affected cells. As the infection progresses, these cells become rounded and detach from each other. Intercellular spaces become wider accompanied by breaking of desmosomal attachments. Destruction of cell organelles and death follows. Such cells slough off the corneal surface creating a depressed area in the center of the lesion. In the meantime, infection spreads to the adjacent cells which undergo the same process of morphological changes.

The lesions produced by HSV, type 2, are raised from the corneal surface in contrast to the flat HSV type 1 lesions (Hollenberg et al., 1976; Hudson et al., 1976; Oh and Stevens, 1973).

HSV particles have been detected in the nuclei (fig. VIII-9), cytoplasm, intercellular spaces of all the epithelial cell layers and on the basement membrane (Takemura and Kitano, 1960; Takemura, 1963; Tanaka and Kimura, 1967; Tanaka and Togni, 1968; Edelhauser et al., 1969; Van Horn et al., 1970; Hollenberg et al., 1976; Hudson et al., 1976).

HSV multiplies in the nucleus from where it passes out into the cytoplasm. During its egress it acquires an outer envelope from the nuclear membranes. Hudson et al. (1976) showed envelopment of a group of virions inside the nucleus. The authors proposed that this phenomenon might be related to the transport of virus.

The development of inclusion bodies in some infected nuclei in our studies *(vide infra)* might be related to the same phenomenon. Van Horn et al. (1970), finding increased cytoplasmic tubules in infected cells, proposed that mature virions might egress out of the cell through these tubules. Schwartz and Roizman (1969) described a similar system in cells infected in tissue cultures.

Van Horn et al. (1970) also measured intracellular membrane

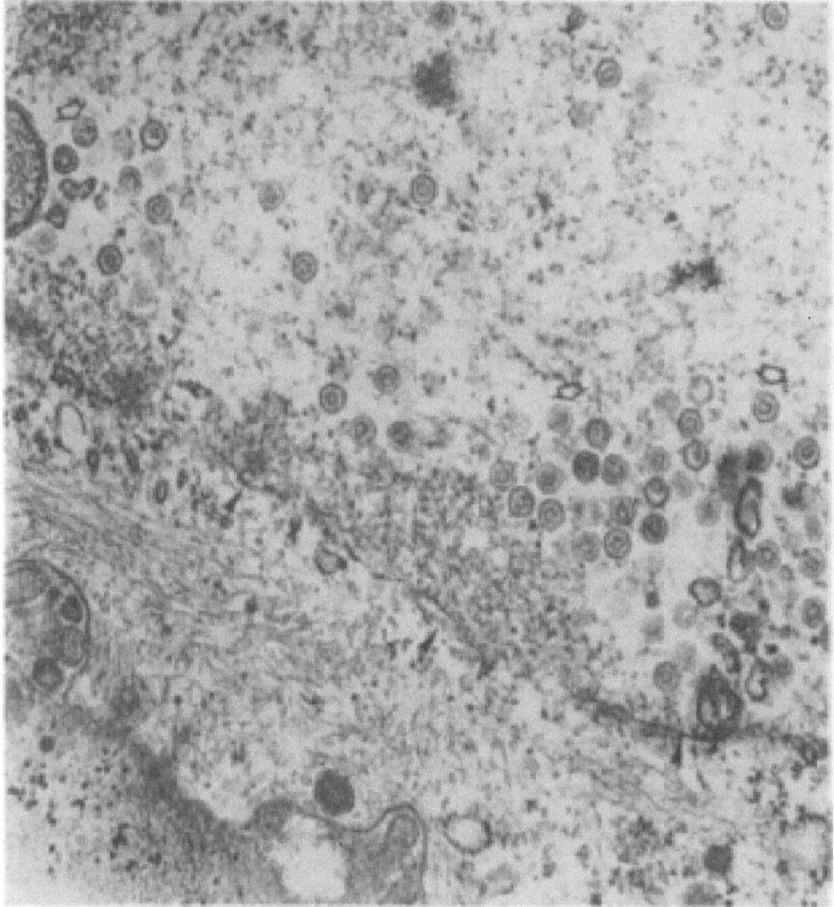

Fig. VIII-9. — Herpes simplex virus particles (empty arrows) in the nucleus of a rabbit corneal epithelium cell. The nuclear chromatin is rarefied and the nuclear membrane is degenerated (arrows). Experimental keratitis. Electron microscopy. × 36 500.

potentials of infected epithelial cells. Already in the punctate lesions the intracellular membrane potentials were lower than normal. These authors ascribed the decreased membrane potentials to membrane alterations resulting in permeability disturbances; so that the cells could not maintain ion concentration differences.

The corneal stroma under the punctate lesions is thicker and contains an increased number of keratocytes with extensively developed endoplasmic reticulum. Van Horn et al. (1970) did not observe any virus particles in the stroma. In experimental keratitis, however, degenerating keratocytes have been shown to contain HSV particles (Tanaka and Kimura, 1967; Tanaka and Togni, 1968; Edelhauser et al., 1969). Dawson et al. (1968) found HSV in 5 of 19 corneal buttons of herpetic keratitis removed at keratoplasty. In another study mature enveloped virus particles were rare in the corneas from 20 patients with chronic or recurrent herpes simplex keratitis (Meyers et al., 1979). The usual finding was naked particles or particles without cores.

Herpes virus antigens however could be demonstrated in the degenerating keratocytes by immunoperoxidase study (Meyers et al., 1979). The authors concluded that a replication of virus in the stroma plays only an insignificant role in maintaining stromal disease whereas the presence of herpes virus antigens could contribute to immune-inflammation in chronic stromal keratitis.

Fluorescent antibody techniques are especially usefull to localise HSV specific antigens in infected cells. Positive results have been reported from 55-82% (Kaufmann, 1960; Petit et al., 1964; Freyler et al., 1976). In experimental HSV keratoconjunctivitis, Uchida and Kimura (1965) found fluorescent antibody staining a better diagnostic method than hematoxylin-eosin staining of scrapings and sections.

Cytology of HSV superficial keratitis

We first reported the replication stages of HSV and the development of disseminating inclusion bodies in rabbit corneal epithelium studied by the corneal replica technique (Maudgal, 1976; Maudgal and Missotten, 1977a and b). The earliest cytological lesion is an enlargement of the nucleolus which may be surrounded by a clear halo (fig. VIII-10a). The pars amorpha of the nucleolus diffuses into the cytoplasm to form "A type" inclusions ("A bodies" of Love and Wildy, 1963). The "A bodies" (fig. VIII-10b) are of variable shape and size and may enlarge to displace the nuclear chromatin to the periphery. "A granules" appear in the "A bodies" which may fill it eventually (fig. VIII-10c). The "A granules" are replicating and maturing virus particles. At this stage, the nuclear membrane of some cells balloons out to release part of its contents enveloped by a thin membrane (fig. VIII-10e). This granular material extends in long chains towards other cells. In doing so, quite often, it forms beaded chains where rounded inclusions of different sizes containing "A granules" are connected to each other by thin filaments. Ulti-

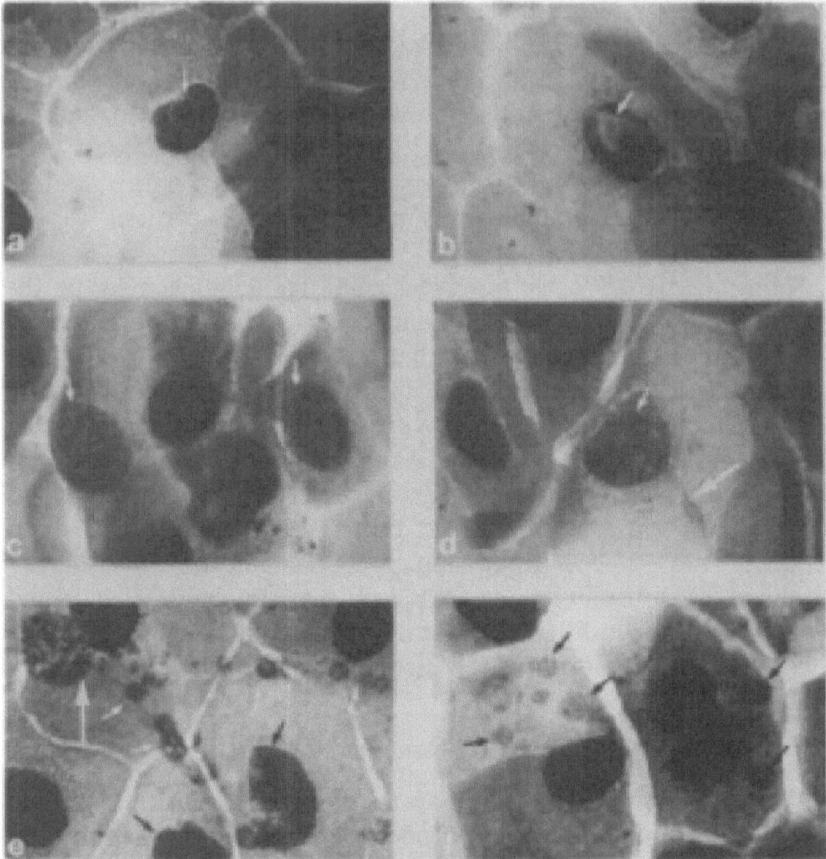

Fig. VIII-10. — Replication of the herpes simplex virus in the rabbit corneal epithelium. Replica technique TBM stain:
(a) Enlargement of the nucleolus surrounded by a clear halo (arrow). × 270.
(b) Arrow indicates an intranuclear "A body". × 270.
(c) Arrows indicate two nuclei filled with "A granules". × 300.
(d) Rearrangement of "A granules" into rounded inclusions in the nucleus (small arrow). Large arrow indicates an extension of filamentous nuclear material released from some other cell. × 300.
(e) Ballooning of the nuclear membrane (large arrow) to release material containing "A granules", which extends in long chains of rounded inclusions (small white arrows) connected by thin filaments. Black arrows point to two nuclei containing "A granules". × 200.
(f) Free rounded inclusions (arrows) disseminate and appear to have affinity for the nuclei of other cells. × 200.

mately the thin interconnecting filaments disappear leaving free rounded inclusions (fig. VIII-10 f). The rounded inclusions show an internal ring structure and may lie inside or outside the cells. Sometimes the rearrangement of "A granules" into rings or rounded inclusions occurs already inside the nucleus before they are extruded out of the cell (fig. VIII-10 d). The rounded inclusions appear to have affinity for the nuclei of other cells as they are mostly located near to the nuclei. We believe that the phenomenon of rounded inclusion formation helps in the transport of the virus from its site of replication. The frequency of development of the "rounded inclusions" is highest in the early stages of infection and gradually diminishes with time.

As the replication of the virus goes on in the nucleus, other cytological changes are occurring in the cell. The cytoplasm becomes much more granular and shows abundance of RNA even in the superficial corneal epithelium cells which normally contain only a little amount of RNA (Maudgal and Missotten, 1978a). Similarly the nuclei show a greater amount of DNA than normal cells. The nuclear chromatin is extruded out into the cytoplasm to form "C-bodies" which disappear by dispersion into the cytoplasm. "C-mitotic lesions" or colchicin-like effect produces multinucleate giant cells (Maudgal and Missotten, 1978b; and 1979a); but their occurrence is infrequent in the superficial corneal epithelium.

In the early stages of infection isolated epithelium cells become rounded and shrunken. With the passage of time their number markedly increases and some of them fuse to form variable sized

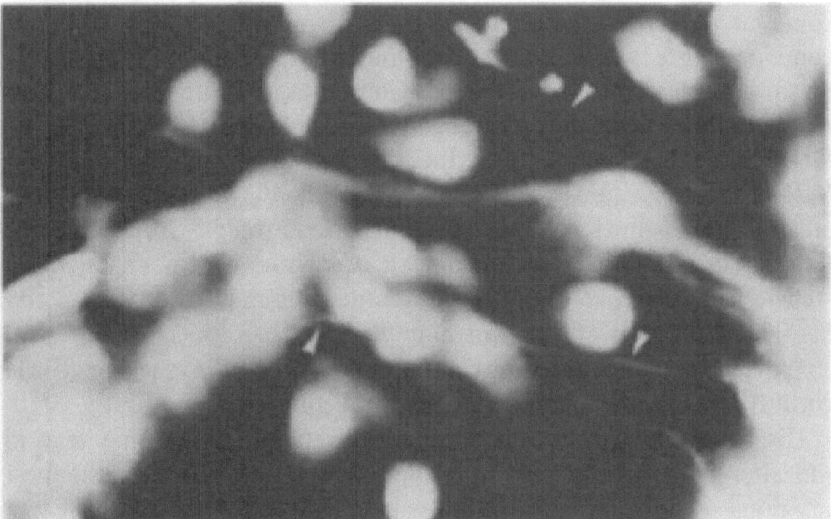

Fig. VIII-11. — Pseudopodia-like processes (arrows) extend from the rounded cells or syncytia. Acridine orange staining. Fluorescence microscopy. × 480.

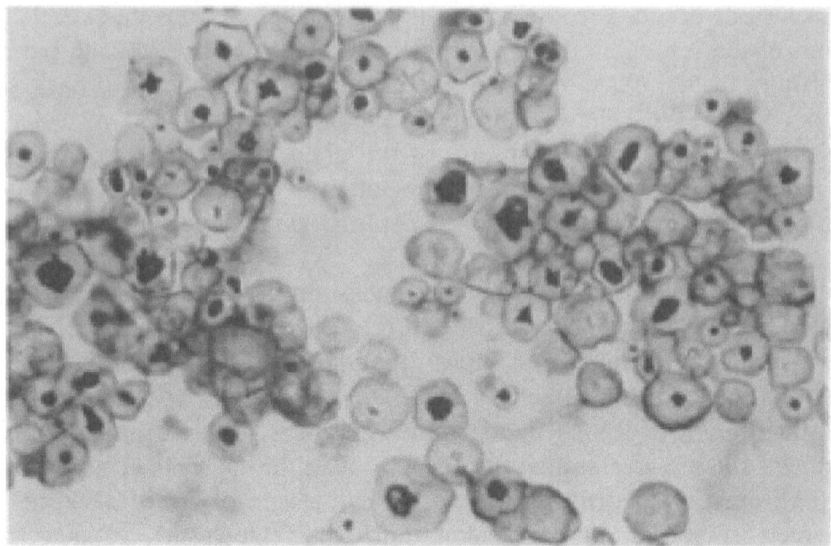

Fig. VIII-12. — Numerous ghost cells in the superficial epithelium. Experimental herpes simplex keratitis. Colloidal iron stain. × 280.

syncytia. The syncytia distincly differ from the giant polykaryocytes containing micronuclei produced by a "C-mitotic" lesion. Syncytia contain bizarre shaped nuclei and nuclear fragments. In the cytoplasm granular DNA particles, probably viral, may be diffusely scattered. Various sized thin pseudopodia-like processes containing some DNA and RNA extend from the syncytia towards other cells (fig. VIII-11). Finally, ghost cells appear after about two weeks post inoculation. The ghost cells are variably sized, roughly rounded cells having eosinophilic cytoplasm and a basophilic central mass, often stellate in appearance (fig. VIII-12). Some cells may be devoid of any basophilic material and appear empty.

We did not encounter any inflammatory cells in the superficial corneal epithelium at any time after infection.

Histochemically there is destruction of reticulin which may lead to the alterations in the cell wall. The changes in the histochemical reactions as compared to normal superficial epithelium indicate the synthesis of virus-specific glycoprotein by the infected cells (Maudgal and Missotten, 1979a).

Replica histology of dendritic ulcers

Study of human herpes simplex dendritic and punctate keratitis by replica technique gave a typical histological appearance (Maudgal and Missotten, 1978b and 1979b). The dendrites and the punctate lesions contain rounded epithelial cells which fuse to form variable sized syncytia (figs. VIII-13 and VIII-14). The nodular areas and terminal

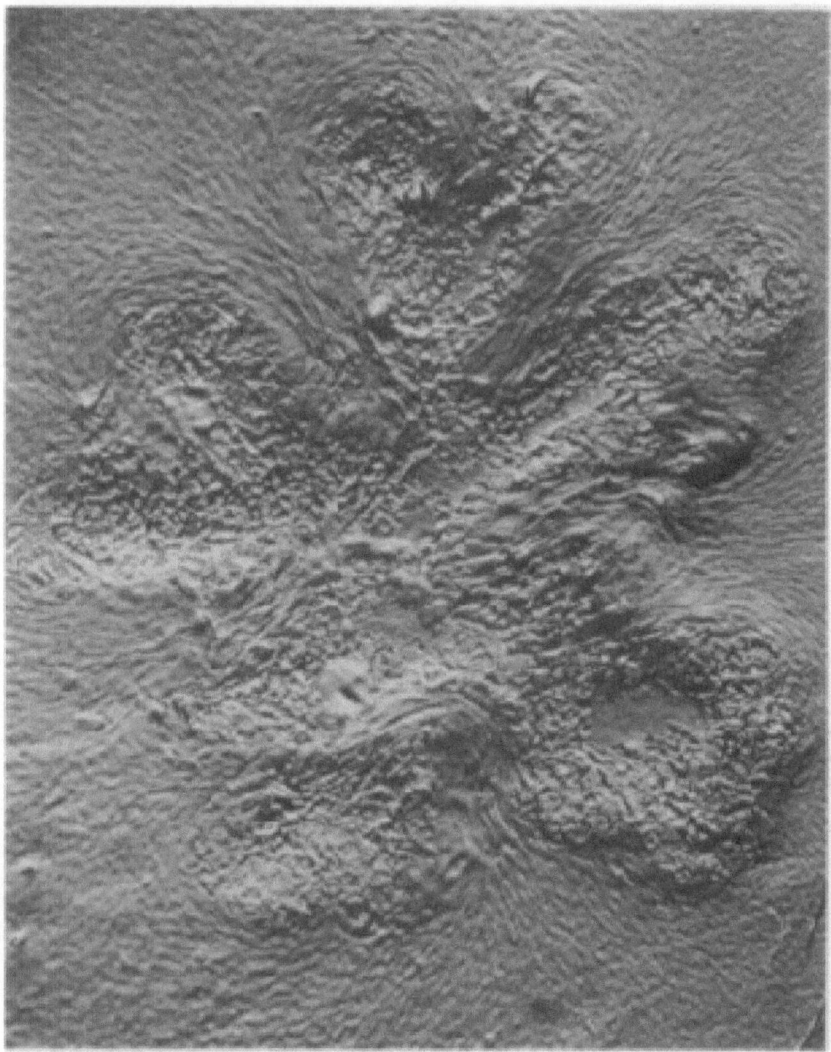

Fig. VIII-13. — Corneal replica of a dendritic ulcer of a patient. Oblique illumination microscopy shows the rounded and fused cells in the dendrite. Elongated cells are present along the periphery of the ulcer. × 80.

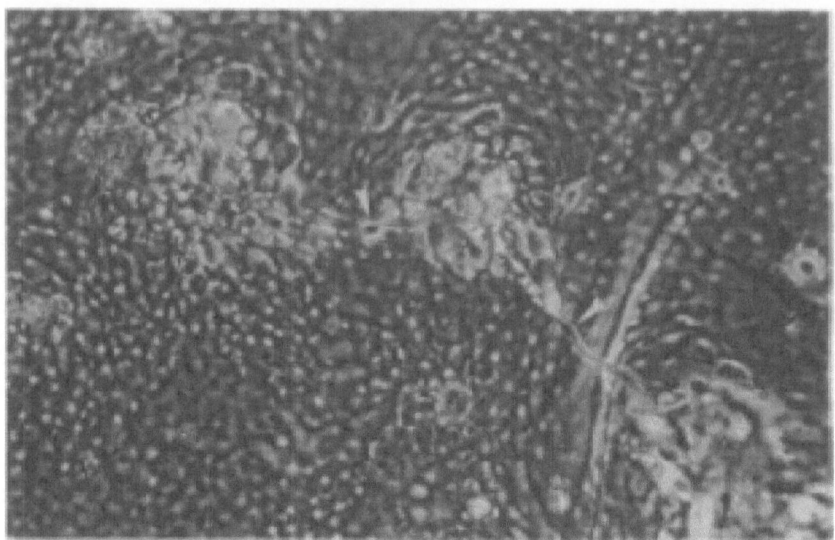

Fig. VIII-14. — Punctate lesions of herpes simplex keratitis are interconnected by pseudopodia-like extensions. Phase contrast microscopy of the replica. ×130.

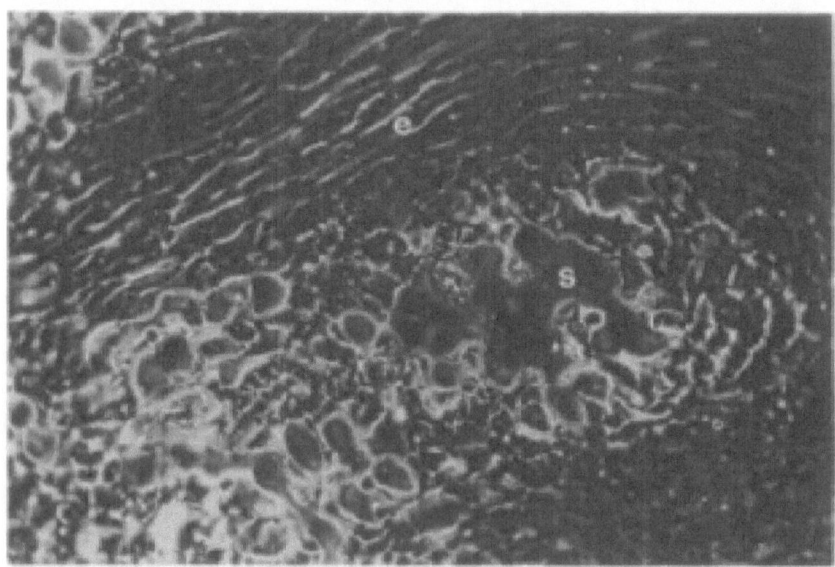

Fig. VIII-15. — Terminal bulb in a dendritic ulcer is surrounded by the elongated cells (e) and contains rounded cells and syncytia (s). Phase contrast microscopy of the replica. ×160.

bulbs of the dendrites contain larger syncytia. Variable sized pseudo-podia like processes (fig. VIII-14) extend from the syncytia to peripheral cells which upon coming in contact with these processes also become rounded and fused. The cytological changes in the syncytia are similar to those of experimental keratitis described earlier but in larger dendrites necrosis of syncytia may be seen. Partly fused cells are present at the borders of syncytia. The dendrites and the punctate lesions are surrounded by a few rows of elongated epithelial cells which run parallel to the long axis of the dendrite or its branches and form an arcuate pattern around the terminal bulbs (figs. VIII-13; VIII-14 and VIII-15).

The elongated cells represent the area of palisading seen clinically around a dendrite. The partly fused cells and the elongated cells show intranuclear inclusions, "A-granules" and deformed nuclei. Cytoplasmic inclusions are rarely seen. Nuclear inclusions and cell edema are present upto about 4 mm away from the dendrites. Clinically such areas appear normal. However, if epithelial bedewing is seen at the slitlamp; the nuclear lesions are found in extensive areas. Like in experimental keratitis we did not find any inflammatory cells in human HSV keratitis except when complicated by secondary bacterial infections. Ghost cells were not so numerous as in experimental keratitis.

Morphogenesis of the dentritic figure

The morphogenesis of dendritic figure, so characteristic of HSV keratitis, has been a matter of speculation and research. It has been assumed that the dendritic figure corresponds to the anatomic pattern of corneal nerve filaments (Fisher, 1933; Baum, 1970a) but this has been conclusively refuted by nerve degeneration studies (Sugiura and Kondo, 1961) and by destroying the corneal nerves by epithelial scraping followed by penetrating autografts in rabbit (Baum, 1970b). The dendritic lesions developed in the absence of any evidence of nerve regeneration.

On the other hand, on the basis of their experimental studies, Sugiura and Kondo (1961 and 1962) and Sugiura and Wakui (1961), have suggested that the dendritic lesions in herpes simplex keratitis can be understood to extend along the dendritic processes of the polygonal cell system of the epithelium; which would consist of melanocytes that have lost their ability to synthesize melanin. Baum

(1970b), however, believes that the polygonal cell population may represent only the variability of a single cell type in the rapidly mitosing epithelial cells and therefore may not be significant in the morphogenesis of the dendritic figure.

Mosaic like branching polygonal patterns appear in the epithelium if the eyelids are rubbed after instilling a drop of fluorescein (Weddell and Zander, 1950; Schweitzer, 1967). The anatomic basis of this pattern is unknown. It is supposed that a similar unknown anatomic structure in the corneal epithelium may be involved in development of herpetic corneal ulcers.

Our histological investigations of HSV keratitis indicate that the morphogenesis of the dendritic figure may not be related to any specific cell system in the cornea or to the anatomic pattern. We have already mentioned that pseudopodia-like processes containing DNA and RNA extend from the syncytia to the peripheral cells which on coming into contact with the tip of this process also become fused to form another syncytium. In this way the dendrite may extend irregularly in the direction of longer pseudopodia. The nodes in the body of the lesion and the terminal bulbs may represent areas of contact between the groups of cells and the pseudopodialike processes. Alternatively, they may be the sites of punctate lesions which have joined together to form dendritic figure. Broadening of the lesion may occur by cell rounding and fusion of adjacent cells as seen around a syncytium.

Treatment

Destruction of the lesion

Elimination of the focus of active virus multiplication in the corneal epithelium, by simple mechanical debridement (curretage), chemical or thermal cauterization and cryotherapy, is one of the approaches in the treatment of HSV epithelial keratitis. These procedures, however, do not eliminate virus from the eye (Kaufman and Howard, 1962; Havener, 1978). Regeneration of the epithelium leads to clinical cure of the disease. The common disadvantage of these methods is that they are painful.

Debridement of the epithelium may be done with a sterile cotton-tipped-applicator, or any sharp instrument like a scalpel blade (Leopold and Serry, 1963; Binder, 1977). Removal of all loosely attached epithelium leads to healing in a much shorter time and was as effective as IDU in some studies (Patterson and Jones, 1967; Whitcher et al., 1976). To avoid the risk of stromal disease epithelial debridement is preferred to IDU therapy if the dendritic lesions are located in the pupillary area. Debridement should be repeated after 4 days if the dendritic lesions persist (Darrell, 1972; Ostler, 1976b; Dawson and Togni, 1976; Havener, 1978). Ostler (1976b) also recommends the use of 4% cocaine to loosen the epithelium before abrasion.

A cycloplegic drug should be applied topically after debridement. A pressure patch should be given and left undisturbed on the eye for 48 to 72 hours. If the abrasion does not heal within this time the pressure patch should be worn longer (Ostler, 1976b). Some authors advise the use of 0,5% IDU ointment 5 times a day after debridement and patching (Hughes, 1969; Laibson, 1973). It is doubtful, however, if the protection against recurrences outweighs the inhibition of the epithelial repair induced by this drug.

Chemical cauterization was practised in order to treat epithelial HSV keratitis before the development of specific antiviral drugs. Iodine, potassium iodide, trichloracetic acid, carbolic acid, ether, ethyl alcohol, silver nitrate, copper sulfate sticks, etc. have been used by different workers (Gunderson, 1936; Kronenberg, 1941; Howard and Kaufman, 1962; Kimura, 1963; Duke-Elder, 1965). Chemical cauterization should not be done if there is associated stromal disease as these agents irritate and enhance the stromal involvement (Havener, 1978). In the opinion of Ostler (1976b) all cauterizing agents produce stromal damage and, therefore, should be avoided.

For the last three years we no longer employ the above mentioned chemical agents and we do not recommend their use. At the most the cotton-tipped applicator used for debridement may be soaked with a minimum amount of iodine alcohol to sterilize the applicator, but not enough to impregnate the cornea.

We have met with considerable success in treating the herpes simplex keratitis by making in vivo corneal replicas (see Chapter I). During the development of this technique we found that the dendritic ulcers of the cornea healed after making the replica (Missotten and Maudgal, 1977; Maudgal and Missotten, 1977b). No deleterious effects of the technique have been observed on the eye during a large number of animal experiments and more than 100 patients with superficial keratitis of herpetic or other etiology. In a recent evaluation of the results on herpes simplex keratitis (Maudgal et al., 1979 a) all the dendrites without or with *minimal stromal infiltrates* healed in 22 eyes in 3-7 days (average 4.4 days) after making the replica. Three recurrences were seen. In one patient the relapse was triggered by upper respiratory tract infection and fever three weeks after the eye had healed on making the replica. Early recurrences within one week were seen in two cases in which the replica was limited to the area of the lesions. Since we found that herpes simplex lesions were also present in cells farther away from the dendritic ulcer (Maudgal and Missotten, 1978 a and b) we now make replicas of larger areas surrounding the ulcers and the early recurrences do not occur.

In a second group of 25 patients *with epithelial and stromal disease* all epithelial dendritic lesions healed within one week but there was no direct effect on stromal disease. Therefore, treatment was continued with IDU to prevent recurrences under antibiotic cover and cycloplegics. Seven patients healed on this regimen in two weeks while in others local corticosteroids had to be added as the stromal keratitis deteriorated. Dendritic ulcers recurred in four patients on corticosteroid therapy. They were treated by a second replica. In one case there was a third recurrence with aggravation of stromal disease. This eye developed perforating corneal ulcer and was treated by keratoplasty. The rest of the patients healed with various degrees of corneal scarring depending on the degree of initial stromal involvement.

Post replica treatment is similar to that after epithelial debridement. Cycloplegics are used only when distinct stromal infiltration is present. The general attitude is to avoid corticosteroids unless the stromal keratitis deteriorates.

All patients in this series had previous unsuccesfull treatment. Local IDU medication, mechanical debridement; chemical, thermal and cyro-cauterization had been tried in different cases. Prompt healing of dendritic ulcers suggests that making a corneal replica is a rather succesful method to treat this disease. It is possible that the embedding of the epithelium in the collodion membrane prevents dissemination of infected cells that might occur in simple mechanical debridement. Another advantage may be that penetration of amyl acetate into the deeper epithelium and superficial stroma fixes the cells. However, recovery from this damage is quick (Missotten and Maudgal, 1977; Maudgal, 1978). In principle, herpes virus should also be sensitive to amyl acetate due to its lipid solvent characteristics.

Thermal cautery, in our opinion, should not be used for destroying the epithelial lesions. As already noted (Chapter III), thermal burns of the cornea are slow to heal.

Cryotherapy or cryocautery of the epithelial lesions has been reported to give good results in HSV infections (Krwawicz, 1965; Bellows, 1966 and 1968; Milverton and Hunyor, 1969; Fulhorst et al., 1972; Tarakji et al., 1978). In other animal experiments and in patients freezing of the epithelial lesions did not produce any better results than other means of therapy (Corwin et al., 1967; Kaufman, 1968; Bellows, 1969; Corwin and Tanne, 1970; D'Alena et al., 1971; Amoils and Maier, 1973; Richards et al., 1977).

Although prompt healing of *epithelial* lesions may be seen after this treatment, cryotherapy has no role in the treatment of *stromal* keratitis and carries a potential risk of permanent endothelial damage (Richards et al., 1977). Repeated freezing of endothelium may lead to intractable corneal edema (Pavan-Langston and Langston, 1975).

Since cryotherapy does not destroy the virus (virologists preserve the virus in frozen media) and because of its potential for endothelium damage we feel that it should not be used for the treatment of herpetic keratitis.

Antiviral drugs

History of antiviral drugs is interesting and not so old. In 1960, Tamm reported that inhibitors of DNA synthesis (antimetabolic drugs) could suppress the replication of herpes simplex virus in tissue culture. However, Kaufman et al. (1962c) first showed that IDU (originally developed as an anticancer drug) was beneficial in the treatment of herpes simplex keratitis. This study also showed for the first time that a viral disease could be treated.

No virucidal drug has been developed so far. The available antiviral drugs inhibit the replication of HSV in the cells so that infection does not spread to the other cells. The already infected epithelial cells fall off as the corneal epithelium is renewed in 4 to 7 days.

IDU (5-iodo-2-deoxyuridine)

Since the original report of Kaufman et al. (1962c), Kaufman and others reported generally good results in subsequent trials in patients and experimental animals (Kaufman et al., 1962a, and 1962b; Kaufman and Maloney, 1962; Perkins et al., 1962; Corrigan et al., 1962; Furgiuele et al., 1962; Hall-Smith et al., 1962; Boyd, 1962; Burns, 1963; Havener and Wachtel, 1963; Maxwell, 1963; Gordon and Karnofsky, 1963; Corwin et al., 1963; Patterson et al., 1963; Jepson, 1964; Laibson and Leopold, 1964; Maxwell and Schliecher, 1964). These studies confirmed the value of IDU despite the findings of some authors that upto 75% spontaneous remissions could occur in the placebo groups (Luntz and MacCallum, 1963; Jepson, 1964). In general it is agreed that IDU cures 55-74% (Coleman et al., 1969; Uchida et al., 1974; Nahmias et al., 1979) cases of herpes keratitis within 10 days as compared to 22-26% of spontaneous remissions in patients (Binder, 1977). IDU administration decreases the virus isolation rates from about 65% in control groups to 4-8% (Coleman et al., 1969; Hollenberg et al., 1976). However, IDU does not significantly change the chance of recurrences compared with placebo, debridement, or proflavine photodynamic inactivation (McGill et al., 1974b).

IDU competitively inhibits the thymidine incorporation into the DNA molecule resulting in faulty DNA chains which are functionally abnormal (Binder, 1977). After infection virus specific thymidine kinase levels increase in the infected cells (Cheng and Ostrander, 1976; Cheng et al., 1979; Prusoff et al., 1979). This enzyme catalyzes the phosphorylation of thymidine which is necessary for DNA synthesis (Cheng et al., 1979). In the presence of HSV specific thymidine kinase in infected cells increased amounts of IDU are incorporated into viral DNA, while very little is phosphorylated in the uninfected cells (Prusoff et al., 1979).

Clinically, IDU 0.1% drops are administered every hour during the day and every two hours at night. Alternatively, 0.5% IDU ointment may be applied five times a day (Kaufman, 1963). We prescribe IDU drops every hour during the day and ointment application before sleep at night for the cases of acute epithelial keratitis. If the dendritic lesion does not respond after 3-4 days of therapy a corneal replica is made. When there is no fluorescein staining of the cornea the frequency of instillation is reduced to 6 times a day and continued for one week. This prolonged treatment is necessary in view of the "rebound phenomenon" of the virus appearance (Havener, 1978).

On topical application IDU penetrates into the cornea poorly (Kaufman, 1963). Its poor penetration, poor solubility and instability in solution (Maloney and Kaufman, 1963; Havener, 1978) are probably responsible for its failure to improve a spontaneous cure rate of about 50% in stromal keratitis (Burns, 1963; Maxwell, 1963; Havener and Wachtel, 1963; Maxwell and Schleicher, 1964; Laibson and Leopold, 1964; Jepson, 1964; Hart et al., 1965).

One advantage of IDU over curettage is that treatment with IDU is painless. However, it is not more effective than curettage in the treatment of epithelial keratitis (Jones, 1967; Jones and Patterson, 1967; Whitcher et al., 1976). In addition IDU suffers from a number of drawbacks. Binder (1977) has summarized the disadvantages of IDU-therapy as follows: IDU is topically toxic and much more so in dry eyes due to increased concentration or decreased dilution; is topically sensitizing, producing drug allergy; causes lacrimal punctum stenosis and obstruction, follicular conjunctivitis, lacrimation, narrowing of meibomian gland orifices, inhibition of keratocyte mitosis, inhibition of corneal stromal repair and a decrease in the strength of healing corneal wounds; and may affect the rate of epithelial regeneration. Prolonged administration may lead to punctate keratitis, subepithelial and intra epithelial edema, and corneal opacities. The side effects of IDU are reversible on discontinuation of medication (McGill et al., 1974b).

IDU should not be prescribed in epithelial lesions of non herpetic origin. Its administration can aggravate a bacterial infection (Yamaguchi et al., 1979). Quéré et al. (1967) stated that the use of IDU in Thygeson's punctate keratitis promotes Bowman's membrane opacities. IDU is not advised after keratoplasty or other corneal incisions (Havener, 1978). Moreover its use is contraindicated in pregnant women because of its teratogenic effects (Itoi et al., 1975).

Vidarabine (Ara-A)

Ara-A (9-β-D-arabinofuranosyladenine; adenine arabinoside; Vira-A) is a nonhalogenated antimetabolite purine derived from the fermentation of filtrates of *streptomyces antibioticus* (Pavan-Langston and Langston, 1975). It was first synthesized as an anticancer drug in 1960 (Lee et al., 1960) and soon demonstrated to have antiviral activity against HSV, vaccinia virus, cytomegalo-virus in vitro (Private De Garilhe and De Rudder, 1964; Freeman et al., 1965; Sidwell et al., 1967) and vaccinia virus in vivo (Sidwell et al., 1968a). Later Ara-A was found to have broad spectrum activity against DNA viruses in vitro and significant therapeutic activity against herpes simplex keratitis in hamsters and against central nervous system infections in mice (Schabel, 1968a).

Ara-A was originally found to be ineffective in the experimental ocular herpes infection in rabbits, where saturated solution of Ara-A (0.06%) was compared with 0,1% solution of IDU (Johnson and Jervey, 1964). Later studies showed that due to its low solubility the concentration of Ara-A was too low. In 0.3% or higher ointment form, Ara-A was effective in the treatment of HSV keratitis in hamsters (Sidewell et al., 1968b). In further studies with hamsters and rabbits topical Ara-A as 0.5% to 20% suspension and 0.3% to 20% ointment was effective in treating herpetic keratitis (Sloan, 1975). It could also be administered subconjunctivally or subcutaneously (Kaufman et al., 1970) but causes irritation and granuloma formation.

A large number of subsequent open and double blind trials in experimental and clinical keratitis have demonstrated that Ara-A as 3.3% ointment is as effective as IDU in the treatment of HSV type 1 and 2 keratitis and also effective in the treatment of IDU intolerant or resistant cases (Pavan-Langston, 1973 and 1975b; Pavan-Langston et al., 1974; McGill et al., 1974b; Nesburn et al., 1974b; Hyndiuk et al., 1975; Laibson et al., 1975; Pavan-Langston and Buchanan, 1976; Niedermeiers, 1976; O'Day et al., 1976; Kaufman, 1976; McGill, 1977). In one clinical double blind study neither Ara-A nor IDU were better than placebo but the difference was not statistically significant (Markham et al., 1977).

Ara-A has been administered intravenously (1 mg Ara-A in 2 ml of 5% dextrose upto 20 mg/kg/day) in the treatment of herpetic keratouveitis (Brightbill and Kaufman, 1974; Abel et al., 1975) without serious toxic effects (nausea, myalgia and temporary hematological changes) but intramuscular injections are not effective; probably because absorption is limited by granuloma formation (Brightbill and Kaufman, 1974).

Ara-A does not penetrate the cornea as such. It is deaminated to hypoxanthine arabinoside (Ara-Hx), a more soluble compound possessing 20% of the antiviral activity of Ara-A or IDU (Pavan-

Langston et al., 1973 and 1974). Penetration of Ara-A is increased after epithelial debridement. Egerer and Drobec (1978) reported healing of the dendritic lesions in an average 2.4 days if Ara-A ointment was applied after abrasion wound was healed. Addition of adenosine deaminase inhibitor (ADAI) increases the activity of Ara-A but not of Ara-Hx and Ara-AMP (Falcon and Jones, 1977).

Ara-AMP (5'monophosphate form of adenine arabinoside) is much more soluble (50 mg/100 ml) and slowly metabolized in humans (Pavan-Langston and Langston, 1975). Ara-AMP is more effective than Ara-A in the treatment of HSV type 1 and 2 keratouveitis (Sidwell et al., 1975, Kaufman and Varnell, 1976). Ara-AMP, however, severely retards epithelial wound healing, and produces pathological changes in the epithelium, stromal edema, cellular infiltration, neovascularization and iritis (Foster and Pavan-Langston, 1977). Therefore Ara-AMP should be avoided in the presence of geographic ulcers, recently transplanted eyes, or eyes with collagenase-like melting problems (Pavan-Langston, 1979).

Ara-A is less toxic to the eye than IDU but superficial punctate keratopathy and punctal occlusion have been described (Hyndiuk et al., 1975). These lesions are reversible on discontinning Ara-A therapy.

Trifluorothymidine (TFT, F_3-TDR)

TFT is a pyrimidine nucleoside like IDU with the difference that iodine atom is replaced by three fluoride atoms (Heidelberger et al., 1964). In experimental and clinical open and double blind studies as 1-5% drops, it was found to be more effective than IDU and equally or slightly better than Ara-A and also effective in cases resistant to IDU or Ara-A therapy (Kaufman and Heidelberger, 1964; Hyndiuk and Kaufman, 1967; Wellings et al., 1972; McGill et al., 1974a; Laibson et al., 1977; McGill, 1977; Pavan-Langston and Foster, 1977). TFT penetrates the cornea better and may be used topically in the treatment of herpetic iritis (Sugar et al., 1973). TFT has no cross allergenicity with IDU or Ara-A (Pavan-Langston and Langston, 1975).

TFT delays corneal wound healing more than IDU (Gasset and Katzin, 1975); it rarely produces topical allergy (Jones, 1975) and punctal narrowing (McGill et al., 1976). When given systemically it is teratogenic but not on topical administration (Dexter et al., 1972; Itoi et al., 1975). Because of its toxicity it can not be administered systematically (Pavan-Langston and Foster, 1977).

Metabolic studies in mice indicate that TFT is hydrolized to inactive compounds 5-carboxyuracil and 5-carboxyuridine (Rogers et al., 1969).

Novel antiviral drugs

Out of other antiviral agents EDU (5-ethyl-deoxyuridine) has recently been shown to be effective in the treatment of experimental herpes simplex keratitis (Gauri and Elze, 1977; Elze, 1979). Although EDU is less toxic than IDU and TFT, comparative studies of its efficacy have not been performed (DeClercq, 1979).

Two other experimental drugs, acycloguanosine (Aciclovir®, 9-(2-hydroxyethoxymethyl)guanine) and BVDU (E-5-(2-bromovinyl)-2′-deoxyuridine) are worth consideration. Both of these drugs are potent and selective antiherpes agents.

Acycloguanosine when applied as 3% ointment in experimental herpetic keratitis in rabbits appears to be as effective as TFT 1% eye drops (DeClercq, 1979). In a recent study acycloguanosine when applied as 3% ointment after minimal wiping debridement was very effective in treating dendritic corneal ulcers of patients as compared to placebo (Jones et al., 1979). In another study it did not interfere with epithelial wound healing (Lass et al., 1979).

BVDU exceeds all other antiherpes drugs in selectivity and potency in tissue culture experiments (De Clercq et al., 1979). Early experiments with BVDU (0.5% ointment) have shown that it is more effective than IDU (0.5% ointment) or placebo in preventing an experimental herpetic keratoconjunctivitis and in the treatment of established keratitis (Maudgal et al., 1980). There was no significant difference in the effect of 0.1% and 2.5% BVDU ointments on the herpetic keratitis in rabbits (Maudgal et al., 1979 b). When applied as eye drops 0.1% BVDU was again better than 0.1% IDU in the treatment of HSV keratitis (Maudgal et al., 1979 b). In selected cases we found BVDU very effective in the treatment of dendritic and geographic ulcers and stromal keratitis resistant to IDU or Ara-A medication. No toxic effects have been noted.

Interferon and interferon inducers

Interferon is a species-specific protein produced naturally by human and animal infected cells or by cells exposed to foreign nucleic acids. It renders other cells resistant to infection by a broad spectrum of viruses (Kaufman, 1972).

In man topical human leukocyte interferon cured more patients and in shorter time when applied after debridement than placebo in a double blind study (Sundmacher et al., 1976). In another study there was no difference in the effect of human leukocyte or fibroblast interferon in the treatment of herpetic keratitis in man (Sundmacher et al., 1978).

Interferon production by the cells can be stimulated in vitro or in vivo by the administration of synthetic double-stranded RNA (polyionosinic-polycytidylic acid, poly I : C or In : Cn). In tissue cultures, the degree of protection was inversely proportional to the viral challenge dose and significantly enhanced by the addition of neomycine (Weissenbacher et al., 1970). Topical or systemic administration of poly I : C prevented the establishement of herpetic keratoconjunctivitis in rabbits. Again the degree of systemic protection was directly related to the serum level of interferon induced (Park et al., 1969). In a double blind study poly I : C resulted in as many cures as IDU in patients (Galin et al., 1976) but it did not prevent recurrences when used prophylactically.

Interferon and poly I : C are non-toxic on topical or systemic administration. However, the effect of poly I : C wanes after a few days even if the treatment is continued (Kaufman, 1972). Therefore, at present it appears useless in the prophylaxis of recurrent herpetic keratitis.

Corticosteroids

Corticosteroids are contra-indicated in the treatment of herpetic epithelial disease. In rabbits corticosteroid treatment of corneas leads to aggravation of clinical disease (Kimura and Okumoto, 1957; McCoy and Leopold, 1960; Kimura et al., 1961) and virus could be recovered for prolonged periods in the corticosteroid treated group than in control group (Takahashi et al., 1971).

The unfavorable effect of corticosteroids in herpetic keratitis has been emphasized by Thygeson (1977). His pre- and post corticosteroid era experience shows that before the advent of corticosteroids herpetic keratitis was relatively benign and self-limited disease but since the advent of corticosteroids the complications of herpetic keratitis have tremendously increased; making it one of the most important causes of blindness in Western countries.

However, in some patients one has to resort to topical corticosteroid therapy in herpetic stromal keratitis as the available antiviral agents are not very effective in curing stromal disease and because these stromal lesions are mainly a delayed hypersensitivity reaction to virus specific proteins (Meyers et al., 1979), even though virus particles can be detected in the keratocytes.

Corticosteroids should be used in the minimum effective doses that would control the reaction, followed by gradual—never abrupt—tapering and cessation (Pavan-Langston and Abelson, 1977). On the other hand, it may be quite difficult to estimate the minimum effective dose for a given patient. Valuable time may be lost if one begins to search the minimum effective dose by starting corticosteroid therapy with dilute concentration, as has been recommended by some authors. In severe cases, we prefer to administer subconjunctival depot corticosteroids (Celestone Chronodose®). We feel that in this way higher concentrations in the corneal stroma can be obtained. If the inflammation subsides, topical dexamethasone 0.1% drops are given and in the case of a favourable response gradually tapered off. However, it is not always easy to stop the corticosteroids as some eyes become corticosteroid dependent.

Thygeson (1977) described a patient who was using local corticosteroids for 25 years to keep his eye quiet. As a general principle, in mild to moderately severe keratitis one should try to avoid corticosteroids and use them only if the inflammation cannot be managed without their use.

Since corticosteroids decrease the resistance of the tissues against infection, topical broad spectrum antibiotics and antiviral agents should be given concomitantly to counter the secondary infections and the reactivation of herpetic epithelial disease. If the epithelial infection recurs corticosteroids should be stopped immediately. In such patients we remove the dendritic lesion by a corneal replica after which the epithelium heals in a few days and resume the corticosteroid therapy afterwards (Maudgal et al., 1979a).

Sometimes patients on corticosteroid therapy, under antiviral and antibiotic cover, deteriorate suddenly and the danger of corneal melting becomes imminent. In the corneal scrapings of such patients we occasionally found an increased number of yeast bodies or candida. These eyes respond well to topical 1% nystatin or flucytosine therapy, 1 drop every hour during day, for 5 to 7 days. This medication can be given concomittently with corticosteroids, antiviral agents and antibiotics.

When no superinfection is detected, corneal melting may be prevented by hourly rinsing therapy (see Chapter IV).

Surgical treatment

Conjunctival flaps, tarsorrhaphy, blow-out patch grafts, corneal adhesives and glued on contact lenses have been tried with some success in the management of herpetic infections unresponsive to medical therapy (Binder, 1977). A conjunctival flap may prevent perforation of a deep ulcer, but will lead to a vascularised scar, interfering with a future keratoplasty. Tarsorrhaphy should be avoided when possible. Glued on contact lenses are not recommended. Bandage lenses may be of some value, but have to be used only under close supervision.

Therapeutic lamellar keratoplasty in the active herpetic disease was enthusiastically advocated at the time when no effective antiviral agents were available. Gradually it became apparent that lamellar grafts did not have any fewer complications than the penetrating grafts. In a recent retrospective study 52% of nonvascularized corneas and 31% of vascularized corneas before keratoplasty had 5/10 or more visual acuity (Colin et al., 1978). Rice and Jones (1973), reported recurrence rate of 65% of stromal keratitis and 35% of epithelial keratitis in their lamellar graft patients within two years of keratoplasty.

The incidence of recurrences after penetrating grafts have been reported from 8.8% to 12% (Hogan, 1957; Ormsby, 1958; Fine, 1958; Rice and Jones, 1973; Fine et al., 1977).

Polack and Kaufman (1972) described 17% early recurrence rate in patients having active herpetic disease before keratoplasty while there were no recurrences in 6 inactive cases. In the series of Pfister et al. (1972) only 44% of the 72 keratoplasties (about two third lamellar) performed for active herpetic disease remained clear with an overall recurrence rate of 18%. Therefore the authors suggested avoiding keratoplasty in the presence of disease activity. Colin et al. (1978) share a similar view that penetrating graft gives best results for post herpetic scarred corneas and that the best choice is to perform surgery after a few months of inactive disease.

On the other hand Rice and Jones (1973) and Fine et al. (1977) did not find any difference in the recurrence rates between the clinically active or inactive disease groups at the time of operation.

In our view, to avoid post operative complications, keratoplasty should be deferred until after a few months the active disease has subsided. Technically, too, it is much easier to operate on a scarred quiet cornea than on an inflamed, thick and vascularized cornea. However, the surgeon does not have any choice except to perform keratoplasty if the cornea perforates. Small keratoplasties (greffe-bouchons) have not been very useful in our hands. A 7 to 8 mm perforating graft within 24-36 hours after perforation presents few technical problems. It always saves the eye and restores good vision in almost half of the cases.

In a nutshell

Epithelial HSV lesions may be treated with antiviral drugs when good patient cooporation is expected. Cooperation may be better when using a new drug, as the opthalmologist unwittingly transmits his feeling about its potency. Mechanical destruction of the epithelium is equally efficient and may result in a faster cure. Local corticosteroid therapy is restricted to stromal lesions. Dosages should be just high enough to suppress immune reaction and should be tapered off very slowly. In case of a sudden deterioration yeast bodies or candida should be suspected. When none are found intensive lavage therapy may prevent surgical intervention.

HERPES ZOSTER

Herpes zoster is an acute infectious disease of man characterized by unilateral segmental inflammation of the posterior root ganglions or of extramedullary ganglions of cranial nerves and a painful vesicular eruption of the skin along the peripheral distribution of the involved nerve (Coriell, 1970).

The Greeks called it "zona or zoster" (meaning girdle) because of the band-like distribution of the skin lesions around the waist. It is also called "shingels" (derived from Latin, "cingullus" meaning girdle) and in Norway and Denmark it is known as "Helvedeslid" (hellfire) because of typical neuralgic pain that follows after the skin lesions are healed (Ostler and Thygeson, 1976).

Etiology

The etiological agent of herpes zoster is the varicella-zoster (V-Z) virus. This DNA virus is morphologically indistinguishable from herpes simplex virus. The transmission of infection occurs by droplet spread (Darrell, 1972) after the infection of respiratory tract. In the non-immune host, usually children, V-Z virus causes chicken pox (varicella) where as in the immune persons, usually adults, herpes zoster (Darrell, 1972; Ostler and Thygeson, 1976). Bokay in 1888 first suggested the possible etiological relationship between zoster and varicella (Coriell, 1970). This relationship is also shown by epidemiology, as the persons exposed to varicella may develop zoster or vice versa.

Epidemiology

Excepting infants who may be protected by maternal antibodies, herpes zoster affects people of all ages without racial differences or seasonal variation (Burgoon et al., 1957; Scott, 1957, Hope-Simpson, 1965; Coriell, 1970). The frequency of infection and its severity and duration increase with age. As most patients are middle aged or older, and often debilitated or suffering from systemic disease (Kass et al., 1952; Burgoon et al., 1957; Scott, 1957), herpes zoster may be considered as an opportunistic infection (Ostler, 1976b). The majority of patients with zoster give a previous history of varicella. Herpes zoster is infectious in the first 2 or 3 days after the appearance of skin eruption (Coriell, 1970). Virus can be isolated during this period from the skin vesicles. Infections in· children are generally less severe, and of shorter duration (Edgerton, 1945; Burgoon et al., 1957). However, manifestations of herpes zoster may be severe and prolonged in patients with deficiencies of immunological system. Kielar et al. (1971) reported such a case in a child who had absent IgA globulines and a delayed hypersensitivity deficiency.

The authors proposed that the immunologic defects may be responsible for the increased susceptibility to varicella zoster infection in children as IgA antibodies have virus neutralizing activity (Tomasi, 1968). A similar hypothesis has been postulated for the increased occurrence of herpes zoster with chronic lymphatic leukemia and Hodgkin's disease in whom gamma globulin levels are decreased (Schanbrum et al., 1960; Sokal and Firat, 1965; Muller, 1967).

Primary or spontaneous cases occur in otherwise healthy people without any precipitating cause (Ostler and Thygeson, 1976). These authors summarized from literature the precipitating stimuli in secondary or symptomatic cases as follows: malignancies, immuno-suppressive agents like the glucocorticoids and irradiation, chronic or severe illnesses as syphilis, tuberculosis, carbon monoxide and arsenic poisoning; and physical trauma.

In some cases, herpes zoster may develop after exposure to varicella or zoster patients. These cases also demonstrate that the two diseases are caused by the same virus. Garrett (1958) reported the occurrence of chickenpox in 4 children after a 3 year old girl with herpes zoster visited the nursery. Berlin and Campbell (1970) described the case of an intern who developed chikenpox 16 days after attending a nurse with herpes zoster. The intern probably transmitted the infection to a renal-transplant patient under his care. This patient was receiving immunosuppressive therapy and developed herpes zoster. One of the patients of Ostler and Thygeson (1976) was an 11 year old boy who developed zoster ophthalmicus with a mild kera-touveitis at the same time when his four siblings developed varicella. This child had suffered from chickenpox one year before, after visiting his grandmother who had herpes zoster. These cases also indicate that the zoster infection may be exogenous.

Rarely zoster infections may recur (Juell-Jensen and MacCallum, 1972).

Pathogenesis

V.Z. virus appears to be transmitted by droplet spread, after respiratory infection. It causes the acute exanthem of varicella in children and nonimmune adults (Darrell, 1972). Virus multiplication occurs at some unidentified site and probably results in intermittent viremia as suggested by the successive eruption of widely spaced lesions (Ribble, 1970).

The zoster eruption later in life may be explained in two ways. According to some, the V-Z virus remains dormant in the dorsal root ganglions after primary infection (Chang, 1971; Ostler and

Thygeson, 1976). However, the virus has been demonstrated only in the skin lesions, although the segmental nerves are always inflamed (Coriell, 1970). Reactivitation usually occurs without any exciting stimuli, but a reduction in host's cellular immunity or pressure on a sensory ganglion from a tumor or trauma may be responsible for recurrence in other cases (Darrell, 1972; Ostler and Thygeson, 1976). After reactivation the virus spreads peripherally to the sensory nerves causing sensory alterations before the eruption of skin lesions. The skin involvement is always limited to the segment supplied by the involved sensory nerve. Sometimes the virus may spread centrally to involve brain and meninges.

The possibility of virus entering the skin or eye and its subsequent migration along the sensory nerves has not been conclusively excluded (Coriell, 1970). Lemp et al. (1974) isolated V-Z virus from the corneal scrapings in superficial punctate keratitis in a 10-year old boy who had neither typical herpes zoster nor was exposed to any clinically evident exenthams.

The authors suggested that at least some corneal manifestations of zoster keratitis may be due to direct infection of the corneal tissues. As already noted the epidemiology of some cases also indicates the possiblity of an exogenous infection.

Clinical manifestations

Herpes zoster ophthalmicus

Involvement of the ophthalmic branch of the trigeminal nerve occurs in 8 to 56% of the herpes zoster cases in different series (Ostler and Thygeson, 1976), and is only next in frequency to thoracic zoster. In aboutg 50% cases of ophthalmic zoster the ocular globe is involved (Coriell, 1970). Almost all cases are unilateral but exceedingly rarely bilateral cases with corneal involvement have been reported (Edgerton, 1945; Walsh and Hoyt, 1969).

After an exposure the incubation period varies from 7 to 21 days. A prodromal phase, with constitutional symptoms with fever, malaise, headache, nausea and pain, paraesthesias or hyperesthesia in the involved nerve dermatome, precedes the eruptive phase by 2 to 5 days. An erythematous dermatitis follows which quickly becomes papular and vesiculated with variable sized groups of vesicles on an erythematous base. The vesicles become cloudy in 2 to 3 days and

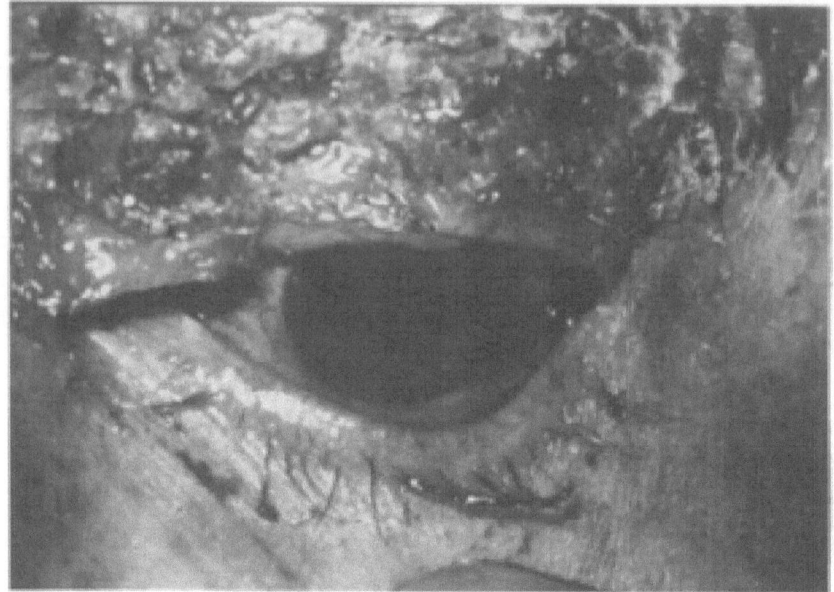

Fig. VIII-16. — Involvement of the upper eyelid in ophthalmic zoster.

crust and dry in 5 to 10 days (fig. VIII-16) (Coriell, 1970). Scarring is common especially if the crusts are removed and if there is associated malignant disease or superinfection occurs (Ostler and Thygeson, 1976). Staphylococcus aureus is the most common secondary invader.

Recently, cases without prodromal symptoms have been reported (Pavan-Langston and McCulley, 1973). On the other hand, rarely, segmentally distributed pain or motor, visceral, or ocular disease may develop without any skin eruption (Ross, 1949; Lewis, 1958). Regional lymphnodes are enlarged and tender early in most cases and rarely may precede skin eruption (Ostler and Thygeson, 1976).

Patient with trigeminal herpes zoster are more likely to develop postherpetic neuralgia (Ostler, 1976 b). The conjunctivitis when present is often papillary but rarely vesicles, pseudomembranes or follicles may develop. Pseudomembranes and vesicular lesions result in scarring (Ostler and Thygeson, 1976).

When the nasociliary branch of the semilunar ganglion is affected, vesicles appear on the tip or side of the nose. This is called the "Jonathan-Hutchinson sign" (Pierce and Jenkins, 1973) indicating an increased likehood of corneal, scleral or ciliary body involvement (Coriell, 1970).

The ocular globe is infrequently involved if the nasociliary branch is unaffected (Doggart, 1933, Edgerton, 1945). Corneal involvement occurs in 50% cases of zoster ophthalmicus and may precede, accompany or follow the eruptive skin lesions (Pavan-Langston and McCulley, 1973).

The early corneal changes vary from mild punctate staining of the epithelium without stromal involvement to severe epithelial and stromal ulceration (figs. VIII-17 and VIII-18) (Edgerton, 1945, Duke-Elder, 1965, Singha and Nirankari, 1970, Darrell, 1972). Most of these changes are considered to be secondary to the temporary sensory denervation of the cornea; but in one study (Hayashi et al., 1973) herpes zoster virus was demonstrated by immunofluorescent technique in 15 of 17 corneal scrapings taken during the first week of disease. Six conjunctival scrapings were also positive. When the

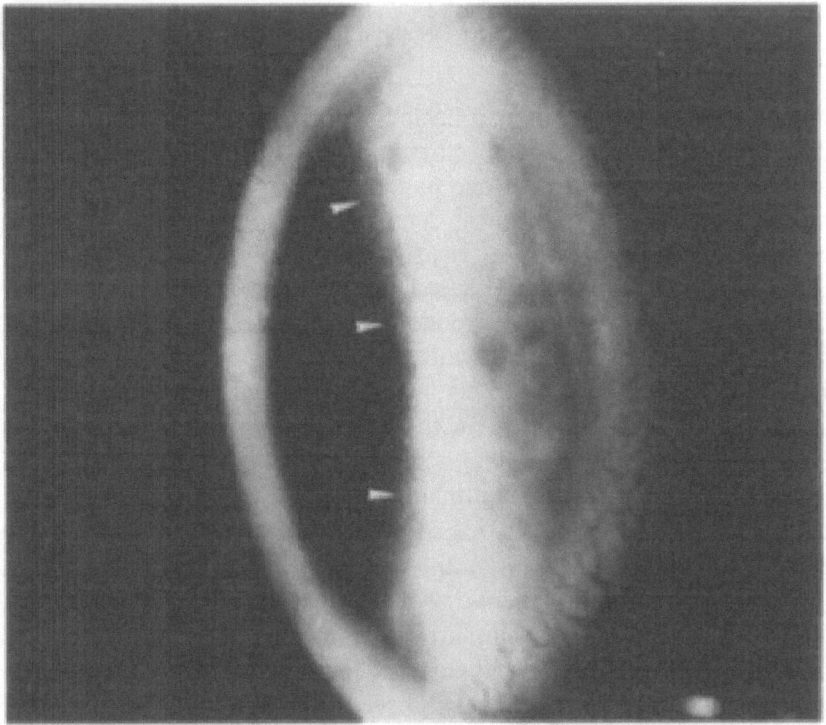

Fig. VIII-17. — Early diffuse punctate keratitis in herpes zoster ophthalmicus visible in retro-illumination (arrows).

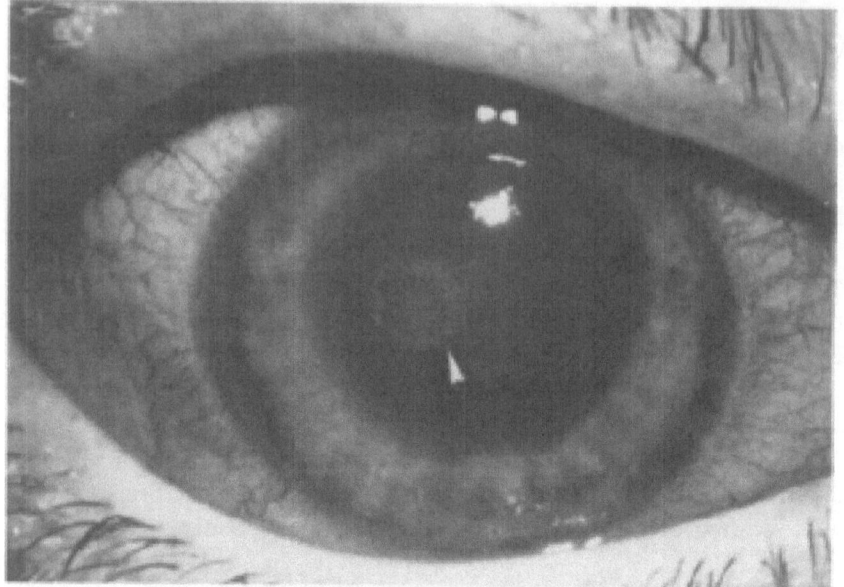

Fig. VIII-18. — Corneal ulcer (arrow) in herpes zoster ophthalmicus.

punctate epithelial lesions had healed spontaneously with subsequent formation of subepithelial opacities, no viral antigens were detected in the corneal scrapings. In one patient keratouveitis recurred after 8 months. At this stage corneal scrapings from the dendritic lesion were again positive for V-Z virus. These findings strongly suggest that the corneal lesions are caused by virus invasion.

Dendritic ulcers have been documented in herpes zoster ophthalmicus by different authors (Kaufman et al., 1963, Acers and Vaile, 1967; Giles, 1969; Sugar, 1971) but attributed to a combined herpes simplex and zoster infection on the basis of their morphology alone. Pavan-Langston and McCulley (1973), however, isolated V-Z virus from three cases of zoster ophthalmicus with dendritic keratitis. The patient of Hayashi et al. (1973) showed the presence of virus in the corneal scrapings by immunofluorescence. Piebenga and Laibson (1973) reported nine patients of herpes zoster dendritic keratitis. Neither V-Z nor herpes simplex virus could be isolated from the corneal scrapings. In five patients tested, herpes simplex antibodies were absent. Recently, we have observed multiple dendritic lesions in a patient (fig. VIII-19) developing 3 months after the initial zoster eruption had healed. The eye was not involved during the initial

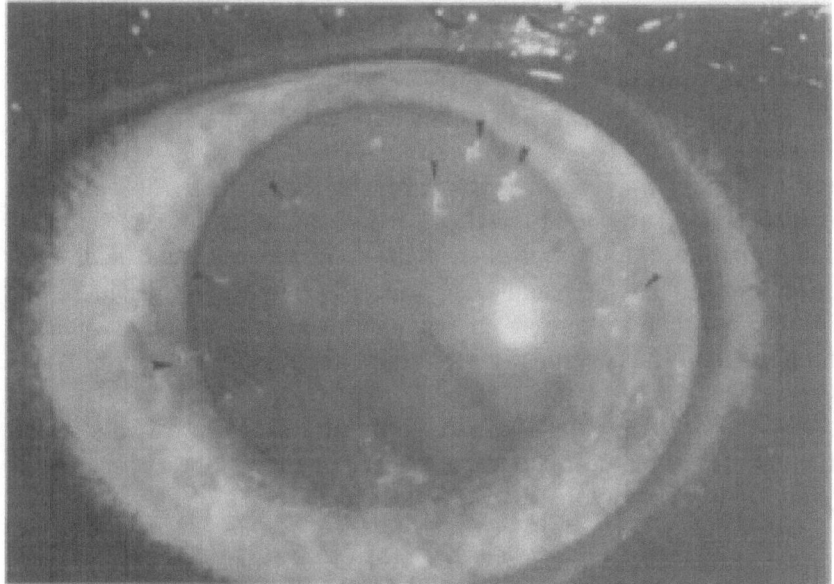

Fig. VIII-19. — Multiple dendritic ulcers arrows in herpes zoster keratitis.

attack. In another patient of dendritic keratitis herpes simplex anti-bodies were absent while V–Z antibodies were present.

The dendritic ulcers of V-Z virus grossly resemble the herpes simplex dendrites, but a discriminating ophthalmologist will see the differences: the zoster dendrite is elevated, stains poorly with fluor-escein and lacks the terminal bulbs characteristic of herpes simplex infection. In our patients palisading of surrounding epithelial cells was also absent. Sometimes, however, herpes simplex dendrite, espe-cially if accompanied by zosteriform skin eruption (caused by herpes simplex virus), may be difficult to distinguish clinically from herpes zoster infection without viral isolation (Forrest and Kaufman, 1976). On the other hand a genuine double infection may exist as con-firmed by V-Z virus isolation from the skin lesions and the herpes simplex virus from the corneal dendritic ulcers (Laflamme et al., 1976). Dendritic keratitis has also been reported in varicella infection (Nesburn et al., 1974 a).

As the epithelial keratitis subsides stromal diffuse, nummular or disciform opacities may develop. Corneal vascularization is common. At present it is not known if V-Z virus is present in these lesions or they are purely the result of antigen-antibody reaction.

Other ocular complications (Ostler and Thygeson, 1976) of ophthalmic zoster are scleritis, anterior uveitis, hyphaema, hypopion and secondary glaucoma. Muscle disturbances due to involvement of III, IV and VI nerve may lead to transitory extra ocular muscle palsies. Involvement of VII nerve may simulate Bell's palsy. Argyll-Robertson-like pupil may occur. Proptosis with extraocular muscle palsy, edema of lids and conjunctival chemosis may mimic orbital cellulitis. Inflammation of the arteries may result in the ischemia of anterior segment with necrosis and destruction. Ischemic changes in retinal vessels may cause retinal edema and exudates or retinal detachments. Hemorrhages and thrombosis of the central retinal vein may occur.

Post herpetic neuralgia is more common in elderly patients affecting about half of the ophthalmic zoster patients above the age of 70 years. It is uncommon in patients below 50 years of age.

Pathology

Giemsa staining of the smears prepared from unruptured vesicles shows multinucleated giant cells and type A inclusion bodies like in herpes simplex infection (Coriell, 1970). Hayashi et al. (1973) described the multinucleated giant cells in corneal scrapings of zoster keratitis but type A inclusions were not seen.

Treatment

Local corticosteroids and mydriatics are the best treatment for zoster keratouveitis (Bergaust and Westby, 1967). Favourable results have also been reported on systemic cortisone or ACTH adeministration (Scheie, 1955; Scheie and McLellan, 1959).

In tissue cultures, IDU interferes with the spread of V-Z virus from cell to cell (Rapp and Vanderslice, 1964). However, IDU is not required in the treatment of superficial epithelial keratitis which always heals spontaneously. It is useless in the treatment of stromal involvement and uveitis which respond to corticosteroids but often need to be used for prolonged periods. On the other hand, IDU must be prescribed if the diagnosis of herpes simplex infection cannot be excluded with certainty. The patient of Forrest and Kaufman (1976) with skin lesions resembling the distribution of zoster ophthalmicus and keratoconjunctivitis was misdiagnosed by different ophthalmologists and treated as V-Z infection until the correct diagnosis of herpes simplex infection was made by virus isolation.

A confusion in diagnosis may also occur in V-Z dendritic keratitis where IDU may be prescribed as a precautionary measure. Two patients of Pavan-Langston and McCulley (1973) were treated with IDU and corticosteroids and the third patient with steroids alone. In any case corticosteroids are not contra-indicated even if dendritic lesions appear during therapy (Piebenga and Laibson, 1973; Forrest and Kaufman, 1976). In one study intravenous cytarabine (ara-c) was reported to give good results in zoster ophthalmicus (Pierce and Jenkins, 1973).

Administration of zoster-immune-globulin obtained from convalescent zoster patients was shown to improve the course of herpes zoster ophthalmicus (Gundersen, 1940). In his series of 22 patients 82% retained 6/18 or better vision who received convalescent blood, whereas only 62% of 39 control patients retained 6/18 or better vision. Gundersen also suggested that if zoster lesions appear on the tip or side of the nose, administration of convalescent serum may prevent the involvement of the eye.

In a double blind study post-herpetic neuralgia was reported to be shortened if systemic corticosteroids were administered for 3 weeks during the acute stage of disease (Eaglstein et al., 1970).

For skin eruption, calamine lotion, 0,25% menthol, and 0,25% phenol can be used to dry the lesions (Darrell, 1972). In our department the skin lesions are treated with application of alcoholic solution of salicylic acid which dries the lesions and prevents secondary infections. Murazyme® ointment is applied locally and also given *per os* in tablet form. To diminish pain didynamic current therapy is given on 10 consecutive days. This treatment prevents the postherpetic neuralgias. If the treatment is started on the first day of eruption the neuralgic pain almost never develops.

To prevent scratching arms of children should be splinted at elbows. In case of secondary infection a broad spectrum antibiotic should be applied locally. Cyproheptadine (Periactin®) has been recommended to prevent severe itching and irritation (Ostler, 1976b). Analgesics like aspirin or codeine may be given to ameliorate pain.

There is no really effective treatment for chronic postherpetic neuralgia (Blaricom and Horrax, 1956). Different vitamin preparations, tranquillizers and sedatives, cortisone, tincture Belladona, diathermy heat and X-ray therapy have been tried without success. Intradermal procaine infiltration is effective in relieving pain but some patients may require avulsion of the portions of trigeminal nerve (Havener, 1978).

BIBLIOGRAPHY

Abel, Jr. R., Kaufman, H. E. and Sugar, J. — Intravenous adenine arabinoside against herpes simplex keratouveitis in humans. *Amer. J. Ophthal., 79,* 659, 1975.

Acers, T. and Vaile, V. — Coexistent herpes zoster and herpes simplex. *Amer. J. Ophthal., 63,* 992, 1967.

Amoils, S. P. and Maier, G. — Cryosurgery and immunotherapy in herpes simplex keratitis. *Brit. J. Ophthal., 57,* 809, 1973.

Bahrani, M. et al. — Generalised herpes simplex and hypoadrenocorticism. *Amer. J. Dis. Child., 111,* 437, 1966.

Baringer, J. R. and Swoveland, P. — Recovery of herpes simplex virus from human trigeminal ganglions. *N. Engl. J. Med., 288,* 648, 1973.

Baringer, J. R. — Recovery of herpes simplex virus from human sacral ganglions. *N. Engl. J. Med., 291,* 828, 1974.

Baringer, J. R. — The biology of herpes simplex virus infection in humans. *Surv. Ophthal., 21,* 171, 1976.

Bastian, F. O., Rabson, A. S., Yee, C. L. and Tralka, T. S. — Herpes virus hominis: isolation from human trigeminal ganglion. *Science, 178,* 306, 1972.

Batignani, A. — Congiuntivite da virus erptico in neonato. *Boll. Oculist., 13,* 1217, 1934.

Baum, J. L. — Melanocyte and Langerhans cell population of the cornea and limbus in the albino animal. *Amer. J. Ophthal., 69,* 669, 1970a.

Baum, J. L. — Morphogenesis of the dendritic figure in herpes simplex keratitis. A negative study. *Amer. J. Ophthal., 70,* 722, 1970b.

Bellows, J. G. — Low temperature treatment of herpes simplex keratitis. *Eye Ear Nose Throat Mon., 45,* 67, 1966.

Bellows, J. C. — Cryotherapy of dendritic keratitis. *Can. J. Ophthal., 3,* 19, 1968.

Bellows, J. G. — Limitations of IDU in herpetic keratitis: cryotherapy as an alternative. *Can. J. Ophthal., 4,* 123, 1969.

Bergaust, B. and Westby, R. K. — Zoster ophthalmicus local treatment with cortisone. *Arch. Ophthal., 45,*787, 1967.

Berkovich, S. and Ressel, M. — Neonatal herpes keratitis. *J. Pediatr., 69,* 652, 1966.

Berlin, B. S. and Campbell, T. — Hospital acquired herpes zoster following exposure to chickenpox. *J.A.M.A., 211,* 1831, 1970.

Binder, P. S. — Herpes simplex keratitis. *Surv. Ophthal., 21,* 313, 1977.

Blaricom, L. S. and Horax, G. — Chronic post herpetic neuralgia. *J.A.M.A., 161,*511, 1956.

Bobo, G. B., Antine, B., Manos, J. P. — Neonatal herpes simplex infection limited to the cornea. *Arch. Ophthal., 84,* 697, 1970.

Boyd, B. F. — Management of herpetic keratitis. Personal interviews. *Highlights Ophthal., 5,* 147, 1962.

Brightbill, F. S. and Kaufman, H. E. — Adenine arabinoside therapy in corneal stromal disease and iritis due to herpes simplex. *Ann. Ophthal., 6,* 25, 1974.

Brown, D,C., Nesburn, A. B., Naugheim, J. S. — Recurrent herpes simplex conjunctivitis. *Arch. Ophthal., 79,* 733, 1968.

Brown, D. C. and Kaufman, H. E. — Chronic herpes simplex infection of the ocular adnexa. *Arch. Ophthal., 81,* 837, 1969.

Brown, S. I. and Weller, C. A. — The pathogenesis and treatment of collagenase-induced diseases of the cornea. *Trans. Amer. Acad. Ophthal. Otolaryng., 74,* 375, 1970.

Buddingh, G. J., Schrum, D. I., Lanier, J. C. and Guidry, D. J. — Studies of the natural history of herpes simplex infection. *Pediatrics, 11,* 595, 1953.

Burgoon, C. F., Burgoon, J. N. and Baldridge, G. D. — The natural history of herpes zoster. *J.A.M.A.*, *164*, 265, 1957.

Burns, R. P. — A double blind study of IDU in human herpes simplex keratitis. *Arch. Ophthal.*, *70*,381, 1963.

Carroll, J. M., Martola, E. L., Laibson, P. R. and Dohlman, C. H. — The recurrence of herpetic keratitis following idoxuridine therapy. *Amer. J. Ophthal.*, *63*, *103*, *1967*.

Carton, C. A. and Kilbourne, E. D. — Activation of latent herpes simplex by trigeminal sensory root section. *N. Engl. J Med.*, *246*, 172, 1952.

Chang, T. — Recurrent viral infection (reinfection). *N. Engl. J. Med.*, *284*, 765, 1971.

Cheng, Y. C. and Ostrander, M. — Deoxythymidine kinase induced in He La Tk⁻ cells by herpes simplex virus type I and type II, *J. Biol. Chem.* *251*, 2605, 1976.

Cheng, Y. C., Hoffmann, P. J., Ostrander, M., Grill, S., Caradonna, S., Tsou, J., Chen, J. Y., Gallagher, M. R. and Flanagan, T. D. — Properties of herpes virus specific thymidine kinase, DNA polymerase and DNase and their implication in the development of specific antiherpes agents. *Adv. Ophthal.*, *38*, 173, 1979.

Cibis, A. and Burde, R. M. — Herpes simplex virus induced congenital cataracts. *Arch. Ophthal.*, *85*, 220, 1971.

Cogan, D. G. et al. — Herpes simplex retinopathy in an infant. *Arch. Ophthal.*, *72*, 641, 1964.

Coleman, V. R., Thygeson, P., Dawson, C. R. and Jawetz, E. — Isolation of virus from herpetic keratitis. *Arch. Ophthal.*, *81*, 22, 1969.

Colin, J., Baikoff, G., Sourdille, P. — La kératoplastie lamellaire dans le traitement de l'herpes oculaire. *J. Fr. Ophthal.*, 1, 501, 1978.

Cook, M. L. and Stevens, J. G. — Evidence that neurons harbor latent herpes simplex virus. *Infect. Immun.*, *9*, 946, 1974.

Coriell, L. L. Herpes zoster. In: *Harrison's principles of Interval Medicine* Wintrose et al. (eds.) McGraw-Hill Book Co. New York, 1970, p. 994.

Corrigan, M. J., Gilkes, M. J., and Roberts, D. S. C. — Treatment of dendritic corneal ulceration. *Brit. Med. J.*, 2, 304, 1962.

Corwin, M. E., Okumoto, M., Thygeson, P. and Jawetz, E. — A double blind study of the effect of IDU on experimental herpes simplex keratitis. *Amer. J. Ophthal.*, *55*, 225, 1963.

Corwin, M.E., Copeland, R. L. and Birnbaum, S. — Cryogenic therapy. *Amer. J. Ophthal.*, *63*, 399, 1967.

Corwin, M. E. and Tanne, E. — Cryotherapy in experimental herpes simplex keratitis. *Amer. J. Ophthal.*, *70*, 33, 1970.

Cowdry, E. V. — The problem of intranuclear inclusions in virus diseases. *Arch. Pathol.*, *18*, 527, 1934.

D'Alena, P., Okumoto, M. and Crawford, B. — Cryotherapy in stromal herpes simplex keratitis in rabbits. *Amer. J. Ophthal.*, *72*, 124, 1971.

Darrell, R. W. — Ocular infections caused by the herpes virus group. In: *Microbiology of the eye*. Locatcher-Khorazo, D. and Seegal, B. C. Eds. Mosby Company, St. Louis, 1972.

Dawson, C., Togni, B. and Moore, Jr. T. E. — Structural changes in chronic herpetic keratitis. Studied by light and electron microscopy. *Arch. Ophthal.*, *79*, 740, 1968.

Dawson, C. R. and Togni, B. — Herpes simplex eye infections: clinical manifestations, pathogenesis and management. *Surv. Ophthal.*, *21*, 121, 1976.

De Clercq, E. — Concluding remarks. *Adva. Ophthal.*, *38*, 297, 1979.

De Clercq, E., Descamps, J., Barr, P. J., Jones, A. S., Serafinowski, P., Walker, R. T., Huaug, G. F., Torrence, P. F., Schmidt, C. L., Mertes, M. P., Kulikowski, T. and Shugar, D. — Comparative study of the potency and selectivity of auti herpes compounds. In: Antimetabolites in Biochemistry, Biology and Medicine. J. Skoda and P. Langen (Eds). *Pergamon Press, Oxford*, 1979, p. 275.

De Voe, A. G. — Medical treatment of acute corneal conditions. *Trans. New Orleans Acad. Ophthal.* St. Louis, C.V. Mosby, 1972.

Dexter, D., Wolberg, W., Ansfield, F., Helson, L. and Heidelberger, C. — The clinical pharmacology of 5.trifluoromethyl-2'-deoxyuridine. *Cancer Res.*, *32*, 247, 1972.

— 140 —

Dohlman, C. H. — The corneal epithelium in disease. XXIII Concilium Ophthalmologicum. Excerpta Medica, Amsterdam, 1979.
Doerr, R. — Sitzungberichte der Gesellschaft der Schweizerischen Augenarzte. Diskussion. *Klin. Monatsbl. Augenheilkd., 65,* 104, 1920.
Doerr, R. and Vochting, K. — Etudes sur les virus de l'herpes febrile. *Rev. gen. Ophtal. (Paris), 34,* 409, 1920.
Doggart, J. H. — Herpes zoster ophthalmia. *Brit. J. Ophthal., 17,* 513, 1933.
Douglas, R. G. Jr. and Couch, R. B. — A prospective study of chronic herpes simplex infection and recurrent herpes labialis in humans. *J. Immun., 104,* 289, 1970.
Duke-Elder, S. — System of Ophthalmology. Vol. VIII. Diseases of the outer eye. Part I. Kimpton, London, 1965.
Eaglstein, W. H., Katz, R. and Brown, J. A. — The effects of early corticosteroid therapy on the skin eruption and pain of herpes zoster. *J.A.M.A., 211,* 1681, 1970.
Easty, D., Entwistle, C., Funk, A. and Witcher, J. — Herpes simplex keratitis and keratoconus in the atopic patient. A clinical and immunological study. *Trans. Ophthal. Soc. U.K., 95,* 267, 1975.
Edelhauser, H. F., Schultz, R. O. and Van Horn, D. L. — Experimental herpes simplex keratitis: corneal hydration, electrolyte content and structural changes. *Amer. J. Ophthal., 68,* 458, 1969.
Edgerton, A. E. — Herpes zoster ophthalmicus. Report of cases and review of literature. *Arch. Ophthal., 34,* 40 and 114, 1945.
Egerer, I. and Drobec, P. — Die behandlung der Herpes-simplex-keratitis mit Vidarabine Augensalbe. *Klin. Monatsbl. Augenheilkd., 172,* 204, 1978.
Ellison, S. A., Carton, C. A. and Rose, H. M. — Studies of recurrent herpes simplex infections following section of the trigeminal nerve. *J. Infect. Dis., 105,* 161, 1959.
Elze, K. L. — Ten years of clinical experiences with ethyldeoxyuridine. *Arch. Ophthal., 38,* 134, 1979.
Falcon, M. G. and Jones, B. R. — Antiviral acitivity in the rabbit cornea of adenine arabinoside, Ara-A-5' Monophosphate, and Hypoxanthine arabinoside; and interactions with Adenosine Deaminase Inhibitor. *J. Gen. Virol., 36,* 199, 1977.
Fine, M. — Treatment of herpetic keratitis by corneal transplantation. *Amer. J. Ophthal., 46,* 671, 1958.
Fine, M. and Cignetti, F. E. — Penetrating keratoplasty in herpes simplex keratitis. *Arch. Ophthal., 95,* 613, 1977.
Fischer, F. P. — Bemerkungen zu Hartinger Artikel über den Zeissischen Cornealreflectographen und seine Hornhautbilder. *Z. Ophthal. Opt., 21,* 65, 1933.
Florman, A. L. and Mindlin, R. L. — Generalized herpes simplex in a 11-day-old premature infant, *Amer. J. Dis. Child, 83,* 481, 1952.
Forrest, W. M. and Kaufman, H. E. — Zosteriform herpes simplex. *Amer. J. Ophthal., 81,* 86, 1976.
Foster, C. S. and Pavan-Langston, D. — Corneal wound healing and antiviral medication. *Arch. Ophthal., 95,* 2062, 1977.
France, N. E. and Wilmers, M. J. — Herpes simplex keratitis and encephalitis in newborn twins. *Lancet, 264,* 1181, 1953.
Freeman, G., Kuehn, A. and Sultanian, I. — Tumorigenic virus and cell responses to biologically active compounds II. Pharmacologic specificity in cell-virus relationship. *Ann. N.Y. Acad. Sci., 130,* 330, 1965.
Freyler, H., Hofmann, H. and Schwab, F. — Diagnosis of herpetic keratitis by immunofluorescence. *Alb. v. Graefes Arch. Klin. Exp. Ophthal., 198,* 155, 1976.
Fullhorst, H. W., Richards, A. B., Bowbyes, J. and Jones, B. R. — Cryotheraphy of herpes simplex keratitis. *Amer. J. Ophthal., 73,* 46, 1972.
Furgiuele, E. P., Pentecost, G. F., Klein, M. and McGavic, J. S. — The effectiveness of IDU in the treatment of herpes simplex keratitis. *Trans. Amer. Ophthal. Soc., 60,* 243, 1962.
Galin, M. A., Chowchuvech, E. and Kronenberg. B. — Therapeutic use of inducers of interferon on herpes simplex keratitis in humans. *Ann. Ophthal., 8,* 72, 1976.
Garrett, F. E. — Herpes zoster ophthalmicus. *Amer. J. Ophthal., 46,* 741, 1958.

Gasset, A. R. and Katzin, D. — Antiviral drugs and corneal wound healing. *Invest. Ophthal.*, *14*, 628, 1975.

Gauri, K. K. and Elze, K. L. — Konzetrationsabhaengige wirksamkeit von 5 athyl-2-desoxyuridin (ADU) bei herpetischen keratitiden in tierexperiment und in der klinik. *Klinik. Monatsbl. Augenheilkd.*, *171*, 459, 1977.

Germer, W. D. — Viruserkrankungen des Menschen. Thieme, Stuttgart, 1954.

Giles, C. — Coexisting herpes zoster and herpes simplex: Ocular involvement. *Eye Ear Nose Thr. Monthley*, *48*, 216, 1969.

Golden, B., Bell, W E. and McKee, A. P. — Disseminated herpes simplex with encephalitis in a neonate. *J.A.M.A.*, *209*, 1219, 1969.

Goodpasture, E. W. and Teague, O. — Transmission of the virus of herpes febrilis along nerves in experimentally infected rabbits. *J. Med. Res.*, *44*, 139, 1923.

Goodpasture, E. W. — The axis cylinders of peripheral nerves as portals of entry to the central nervous system for the virus of herpes simplex in experimentally infected rabbits. *Amer. J. Pathol.*, *1*, 11, 1925a.

Goodpasture, E. W. — The pathways of infection of the central nervous system in herpetic encephalitis of rabbits contracted by contact, with a comparative comment on medullary lesions in a case of human poliomyelitis. *Amer. J. Pathol.*, *1*, 29, 1925b.

Goodpasture, E. W. — Herpetic infections with special reference to involvement of the nervous system. *Medicine (Baltimore)*, *7*, 223, 1929.

Gordon, D. M. and Karnofsky, D. A. — Chemotherapy of herpes simplex keratitis. *Amer. J. Ophthal.*, *55*, 229, 1963.

Grüter, W. — Experimentelle und klinische Untersuchungen uber den Sog. Herpes corneae. *Klin. Monatsbl. Augenheilkd.*, *65*, 398, 1920a.

Grüter, W. — Experimentelle und klinische Untersuchungen uber den sogenaunten Herpes corneae. *Ber. Dtsch. Ophthal. Ges.*, *42*, 162, 1920b.

Gundersen, T. — Herpes corneae, with special reference to its treatment with strong solutions of iodine. *Arch. Ophthal.*, *15*, 225, 1936.

Gundersen, T. — Convalescent blood for treatment of herpes zoster ophthalmicus. Second report. *Trans. Amer. Ophthal. Soc.*, *38*, 124, 1940.

Haas, G. M. — Hepato-adrenal necrosis with intranuclear inclusion bodies. Report of a case. *Amer. J. Path.*, *11*, 127, 1935.

Hagler, W. S., Walters, P. V. and Nahmias, A. J. — Ocular involvement in neonatal herpes simplex virus infection. *Arch. Ophthal.*, *82*, 169, 1969.

Hall-Smith, S. P., Corrigan, M. J. and Gilkes, M. J. — Treatment of herpes simplex with 5-iodo-2-Deoxyuridine. *Brit. Med. J.*, *2*, 1515, 1962.

Hanna, L., Jawetz, E. and Coleman, V. R. — Studies on herpes simplex. VIII The significance of isolating herpes simplex virus from the eye. *Amer. J. Ophthal.*, *43*, 126, 1957.

Hart, D. R. L., Brightman, V. J. F., Readshaw, G. G., Porter, G. T. J. and Tully, M. J. — Treatment of human herpes simplex keratitis with idoxuridine. *Arch. Ophthal.*, *73*, 623, 1965.

Havener, W. H. and Wachtel, J. — IDU therapy of herpetic keratitis. *Amer. J. Ophthal.*, *55*, 234, 1963.

Havener, W. H. — Ocular pharmacology. C. V. Mosby Co, St. Louis, 1978.

Hayashi, K., Uchida, Y. and Ohshima, M. — Fluorescent antibody study of herpes zoster keratitis. *Amer. J. Ophthal.*, *75*, 795, 1973.

Heidelberger, C., Parsons, D. G. and Remy, D. C. — Synthesis of 5-trifluoromethylfluracil and 5-trifluoromethyl-2-deoxyuridine. *J. Med. Chem.*, *7*,1, 1964.

Hogan, M. J. — Corneal transplantation in the treatment of herpetic disease of the cornea.*Amer. J. Ophthal.*, *45*, 147, 1957.

Hollenberg, M. J., Wilkie, J. S., Hudson, J. B. and Lewis, B. J. — Lesions produced by human herpes viruses 1 and 2. Morphological feactures in rabbits corneal epithelium. *Arch. Ophthal.*, *94*, 127, 1976.

Hope-Simpson, R. E. — The nature of herpes zoster: a long-term study and a new hypothesis. *Proc. Royal Soc. Med.*, *58*, 9, 1965.

Howard, G. M. and Kaufman, H. E. — Herpes simplex keratitis. *Arch. Ophthal.*, *67*, 373, 1962.

Howard, R. O. — Herpes simplex keratoconjunctivitis. *Amer. J. Ophthal.,* *62,* 907, 1966.

Hudson, J. B., Hollenberg, M. J., Wilkie, J. S. and Lewis, B. J. — Ultrastructural study of lesions induced in rabbit cornea by herpes simplex virus type 1 and 2. *J. Infect. Dis., 133,* 367, 1976.

Hughes, W. F. — Treatment of herpes simplex keratitis. A review. *Amer. J. Ophthal., 67,* 313, 1969.

Hutchison, D. S., Smith, R. E. and Haughton, P. B. — Congenital herpetic keratitis. *Arch. Ophthal., 93,* 70, 1975.

Hyndiuk, R. and Kaufman, G. E. — Newer compounds in therapy of herpes simplex keratitis. *Arch. Ophthal., 78,* 600, 1967.

Hyndiuk, R. A., Hull, D. S., Schultz, R. O. et al. — Adenine arabinoside in IDU unresponsive and IDU intolerant herpetic keratitis. *Amer. J. Ophthal., 79,* 655, 1975.

Itoi, M., Gnadinger, M. C., Slansky, H. H., Freeman, M. I. and Dohlman, C. H. — Collagenase in the cornea. *Exp. Eye Res., 8,* 369, 1969.

Itoi, M., Gefter, J., Kaneko, N., Ishii, Y., Ramer, R. and Gasset, A. — Teratogenicities of Ophthalmic drugs. *Arch. Ophthal., 93,* 46, 1975.

Jepson, C. N. — Treatment of herpes simplex of the cornea with IDU: A double blind study. *Amer. J. Ophthal., 57,* 213, 1964.

Johnson, A. W. and Jervey, E. D. — Adenine arabinoside and 5-mercaptouracil in herpes keratitis. *Arch. Ophthal., 72,* 826, 1964.

Jones, B. R. — Prospects in treating viral disease of the eye. *Trans. Ophthal. Soc. U.K., 87,* 537, 1967.

Jones, B. R. and Patterson, A. — The management of ocular herpes. *Trans. Ophthal. Soc. U.K., 87,* 59, 1967.

Jones, B. R. — Rational regimen of administration of antivirals. *Trans. Amer. Acad. Ophthal. Otolaryngol., 79,* 104, 1975.

Jones, B. R., Coster, D. J., Fison, P. N., Thompson, G. M., Cobo, L. M. and Falcon, M. G. — Efficacy of acycloguanosine (Wellcome 2480) against herpes simplex corneal ulcers. *Lancet, 1,* 243, 1979.

Juell-Jensen, B. E. and MacCallum, F. O. — Herpes simplex, varicella, and Zoster. J. B. Lippincott Co Philadelphia, 1972.

Kass, E. H., Aycock, R. R. and Finland, M. — Clinical evaluation of aureomycin and chloramphenicol in herpes zoster. *N. Engl. J. Med., 246,* 167, 1952.

Kaufman, H. E. — The diagnosis of corneal herpes simplex infection by fluorescent antibody staining. *Arch. Ophthal., 64,* 382, 1960.

Kaufman, H. E. and Maloney, E. D. — Experimental herpes simplex keratitis. *Amer. J. Ophthal., 66,* 125, 1961.

Kaufman, H. E. — Clinical cure of herpes simplex keratitis by 5-iodo-2-Deoxyuridine. *Proc. Soc. Exp. Biol. Med., 109,* 251, 1962.

Kaufman, H. E., and Howard, G. M. — Therapy of experimental herpes simplex keratitis. *Invest. Ophthal., 1,* 561, 1962.

Kaufman, H. E. and Maloney, E. D. — IDU and hydrocortisone in experimental herpes simplex keratitis. *Arch. Ophthal., 68,* 396, 1962.

Kaufman, H. E., Martola, E. L. and Dohlman, C. — Use of 5-iodo-2-deoxyuridine (IDU) in treatment of herpes simplex keratitis. *Arch. Ophthal., 68,* 235, 1962a.

Kaufman, H. E., Maloney, E. D. and Nesburn, A. B. — Comparison of specific antiviral agents in herpes simplex keratitis. *Invest. Ophthal., 1,* 686, 1962b.

Kaufman, H. E., Nesburn, A. B. and Maloney, E. D. — IDU therapy of herpes simplex. *Arch. Ophthal., 67,* 583, 1962c.

Kaufman, H. E. — Chemotherapy of herpes keratitis. *Invest. Ophthal., 2,* 205, 1963.

Kaufman, H., Dohlman, C. H. and Martola, E. L. — Herpes simplex treatment with IDU and corticosteroids. *Arch. Ophthal., 69,* 468, 1963.

Kaufman, H. E. — Epithelial erosion syndrome: metaherpetic keratitis. *Amer. J. Ophthal., 57,* 983, 1964.

Kaufman, H. E. and Heidelberger, C. — Therapeutic antiviral action of 5-trifluoromethyl-2-deoxyuridine. *Science, 145,* 585, 1964.

Kaufman, H. E., Brown, D. C. and Ellison, E. M. — Recurrent herpes in rabbit and man. *Science, 156,* 1628, 1967.

— 143 —

Kaufman, H. E. — Cryotherapy of herpetic keratitis. *J. Cryo. Surg.*, *3*, 199, 1968.
Kaufman, H. E., Brown, D. C. and Ellison, E. M. — Herpes virus in the lacrimal gland and conjunctiva. *Amer. J. Ophthal.*, *65*, 32, 1968.
Kaufman, H. E., Ellison, E. D. and Townsend, W. M. — The chemotherapy of herpes iritis with adenine arabinoside and cytarabine. *Arch. Ophthal.*, *84*, 783, 1970.
Kaufman, H. E. — Medical treatment of herpes. *Isr. J. Med. Sci.*, *8*, 1231, 1972.
Kaufman, H. E. — Ocular antiviral therapy in perspective. *J. infect. Dis.*, *133* (suppl.), A 96, 1976.
Kaufman, H. E. and Varnell, E. D. — Effect of 9-β-D-Arabino-furanosyladenine 5'-monophosphate and 9-β-D-Arabine furanosylhypoxanthine 5'-monophosphate on experimental herpes simplex keratitis. *Antimicr. Agents Chemother.*, *10*, 885, 1976.
Kibrick, S. and Gooding, G. — Pathogenesis of infections with herpes simplex virus with special reference to the nervous system. In: Slow, temperate and latent viral infections, N.I.N.D.B. Monograph 2, Bethesda, Md. 1965.
Kielar, R. A., Cunningham, G. C. and Gerson, K. L. — Occurrence of herpes zoster ophthalmicus in a child with absent immunoglobulin A and deficiency of delayed hypersensitivity. *Amer. J. Ophthal.*, *72*, 555, 1971.
Kimura, S. J. and Okumoto, M. — The effect of corticosteroids on experimental herpes simplex keratoconjunctivitis in the rabbit. *Amer. J. Ophthal.*, *43*, 131, 1957.
Kimura, S. J., Bonnet, V., Okumoto, M. and Hogan, M. — The effect of corticosteroid hormones on experimental herpes simplex keratitis. *Amer. J. Ophthal.*, *51*, 945, 1961.
Kimura, S. J. — Herpes simplex keratitis. In: infectious diseases of the conjunctiva and cornea. Symposium of the New Orleans Academy of Ophthalmology. St. Louis. Mosby Company, 1963.
Knotts, F. B., Cook, M. L. and Stevens, J. G. — Latent herpes simplex virus in the central nervous system of rabbits and mice. *J. Exp. Med.*, *138*, 740, 1973.
Kronenberg. B. — Treatment of herpetic keratitis with ether. *Arch. Ophthal.*, *26*, 247, 1941.
Krwawicz, T. — Cryogenic treatment of herpes simplex keratitis. *Brit. J. Ophthal.*, *49*, 37, 1965.
Laflamme, M. Y., Kurstak, C., Kurstak, E. and Moriset, R. — Zona ophtalmique et kératite dendritique. *Canad. J. Ophthal.*, *11*, 217, 1976.
Laibson, P. R. and Leopold, I. H. — An evaluation of double-blind IDU therapy in 100 cases of herpetic keratitis. *Trans. Amer. Acad. Ophthal. Otolaryngol.*, *68*, 22, 1964.
Laibson, P. R. and Kibrick, S. — Reactivation of herpetic keratitis by epinephrine in rabbit. *Arch. Ophthal.*, *75*, 254, 1966.
Laibson, P. R. and Kibrick, S. — Reactivation of herpetic keratitis in rabbit. II Repeated reactivations in the same host. *Arch. Ophthal.*, *77*, 244, 1967.
Laibson, P. R. and Kibrick, S. — Recurrence of herpes simplex virus in rabbit eyes: Results of a three year old study. *Invest. Ophthal.*, *8*, 346, 1969.
Laibson, P. R. — Current therapy of herpes simplex virus infection of the cornea. *Int. Ophthal. Clin.*, *13*, 39, 1973.
Laibson, P. R., Hyndiuk, R., Krachmer, J. H. and Schultz, R. O. — ARA-A and IDU-therapy of human superficial herpetic keratitis. *Invest. Ophthal.*, *14*, 762, 1975.
Laibson, P. R., Arentsen, J. J., Mazzanti, W. D., Eiferman, R. A. — Double controlled comparison of IDU and trifluorthymidine in thirty-three patients with superficial herpetic keratitis. *Trans. Amer. Ophthal. Soc.*, *75*, 316, 1977.
Langvad, A. and Voigt, J. — Herpes generalisator infantum. *Dan. Med. Bull.*, *10*, 153, 1963.
Lanier, J. D. — Marginal herpes simplex keratitis. *Ophthal. Digest*, March, 1976.
Lass, J. H., Pavan-Langston, D. and Park, N. H. — Aciclovir and corneal wound healing. *Amer. J. Ophthal.*, *88*, 102, 1979.
Lee, W. W., Benitez, A., Goodman, L. and Baker, B. R. — Potential anticancer agents. XL. Synthesis of the B-anomer of 9-(D-arabinofuranosyl)-adenine. *J. Amer. Chem. Soc.*, *82*, 2648, 1960.

Lemp, M. A., Chambers Jr. R. W. and Lundy, J. — Viral isolate in superficial punctate keratitis. *Arch. Ophthal., 91,8, 1974.*

Lennartz, H. — Diagnosis of herpes simplex. *Adv. Ophthal., 38,17, 1979.*

Leopold, I. H. and Serry, T. W. — Epidemiology of herpes simplex keratitis. *Invest. Ophthal., 2,* 498, 1963.

Lerche, W., Domarus, D. V., Hanke, C., Maass, C. and Gauri, K. K. — Electron microscope studies following treatment with 5-ethyl-2'-deoxyuridine. *Adv. Ophthal., 38,* 49, 1979.

Lewis, G. W. — Zoster sine herpete. *Br. Med. J., 2,* 418, 1958.

Lindgren, K. M., Douglas. R. G. Jr. and Couch, R. B. — Significance of herpes virus hominis in respiratory secretions of man. *N. Engl. J. Med., 278,* 517, 1968.

Lipschutz, B. L. — Untersuchungen uber die Atiologie der Krankheiten der herpesgruppe : Herpes zoster, Herpes genitalis, herpes febralis. *Arch. Derm. und Syph. Berlin, 136,* 428. 1921.

Locatcher-Khorazo, D. and Seegal, B. C. — Microbiology of the eye. C. V. Mosby, St. Louis, 1972.

Love, R. and Wildy, P. — Cytochemical studies of the nucleoproteins of Hela cells infected with herpes virus. *J. Cell Biology, 17,* 237, 1963.

Lowenstein, A. — Atiologische Untersuchungen uber den fieberhaten Herpes. *Munch. Med. Wochenschr., 66,* 769, 1919.

Luntz, M. H. and McCallum, F. O. — Treatment of herpes simplex keratitis with 5-iodo-2'-deoxyuridine. *Brit. J. Ophthal., 47,* 449, 1963.

McCallum, F. O. — Generalized herpes simplex in the neonatal period. *Acta Virol. (suppl), 3,* 17, 1959.

McCoy, G. and Leopold, I. H. — Simplex infections of the cornea. *Amer. J. Ophthal., 49,* 1355, 1960.

McCulley, J. P., Slansky, H. H., Pavan-Langston, D. and Dohlman, C. H. — Collagenolytic activity in experimental herpes simplex keratitis. *Arch. Ophthal., 84,* 516, 1970.

McGill, J., Holt-Wilson, A., McKinnon, J., Williams, H. and Jones, B. — Some aspects of the clinical use of trifluorothymidine in the treatment of herpetic ulceration of the cornea. *Trans. Ophthal. Soc. U.K., 94,* 342, 1974a.

McGill, J., Williams, H., Mc. Kinnon, J., Holt-Wilson, A. D. and Jones, B. R. — Reassessment of idoxuridine therapy of herpetic keratitis. *Trans. Ophthal. Soc. U.K., 94,* 542, 1974b.

McGill, J., Fraunfelder, F. T. and Jones, B. R. — Current and proposed management of ocular herpes simplex. *Surv. Ophthal., 20,* 358, 1976.

McGill, J. — Drug resistance and antiviral agents. Letter. *J. Antimicrob. Chemother., 3,* 284, 1977.

Maloney, E. D. and Kaufman, H. E. — Antagonism and toxicity of IDU by its degradation products. *Invest. Ophthal., 2,* 55, 1963.

Markham, R. H. C., Carter, C., Scobie, M. A. et al. — Double-blind clinical trial of adenine arabinoside and idoxuridine in herpetic corneal ulcers. *Trans. Ophthal. Soc. U.K., 97,* 333, 1977.

Maudgal, P. C. and Missotten, L. — Development of disseminating inclusion bodies in primary experimental herpes simplex keratitis. *Bull. Soc. Belge Ophthal., 179,* 25, 1977 a.

Maudgal, P. C. and Missotten, L. — La réplique de la cornée appliquée à l'étude de la kératite herpétique. *Bull. Soc. Belge d'Ophtal., 175,* 26, 1977 b.

Maudgal, P. C. — The epithelial response in keratitis sicca and keratitis herpetica (an experimental and clinical study). Doctoral thesis, University of Leuven, 1976. *Doc. Ophthal., 45,* 223, 1978.

Maudgal, P. C. and Missotten, L. — Histology and histochemistry of the normal superficial corneal epithelium of rabbit. *Alb. v. Graefes Arch. klin. exp. Ophthal., 205,* 167, 1978a.

Maudgal, P. C. and Missotten, L. — Histopathology of the human superficial herpes simplex keratitis. *Brit. J. Ophthal., 62,* 46, 1978b.

Maudgal, P. C. and Missotten, L. — Histopathology and histochemistry of the superficial corneal epithelium in experimental herpes simplex keratitis. *Alb. v. Graefs Arch. exp. klin. Ophthal., 209,* 239, 1979 a.

Maudgal, P.C. and Missotten, L. — Histopathological study of the human herpes simplex dendritic and punctate keratitis by replica technique. *Docum. Ophthal. Proc. Series, 20*, 211, 1979a.

Maudgal, P.C., Van Deuren, H. and Missotten, L. — Therapeutic effect of corneal replica in herpetic keratitis. *Bull. Soc. Belge d'Ophthal., 184*, 1979a.

Maudgal, P.C., De Clercq, E., Deschamps, J. and Missotten, L. — Evaluation of BVDU for the treatment of experimental herpes simplex keratitis. *Bull. Soc. Belge d'Ophthal. 186*, 109, 1979b.

Maudgal, P.C., De Clercq, E., Deschamps, J., Missotten, L. et al. — (E)-5-(2-bromo-vinyl)-2'-dioxyuridine in the treatment of experimental herpes simplex keratitis. *Antimicrob. Agents Chemother. 17*, 8, 1980.

Maxwell. E. — Treatment of herpes keratitis with 5-iodo-2'-deoxyuridine. *Amer. J. Ophthal., 56*, 571, 1963.

Maxwell, E. and Schliecher, J.B. — Experimental and clinical experiences with IDU. *Eye Ear Throat Month., 43*, 39, 1964.

May, G., Dahn, R. and Rauss, K. — Herpes simplex virus as a cause of encephalitis. *Ger. Med. Mon., 12*, 377, 1967.

Meyers, R.L., Chitjian, P.A. and Fiorello, P. — Studies on immunopathogenesis of chronic and recurrent herpes simplex virus keratitis in man: immunoperoxidase antiboidy study. XXIII, Concilium ophthalmologica Acta Pars II, Excerpta Medica, Amsterdam, 1979.

Milverton, E.J. and Hunyor, A.B.L. — Cryotherapy for dendritic keratitis. *Med. J. Amst., 56*, 889, 1969.

Mintsioulis, G., Dawson, C.R., Oh, J.O. and Briones, O. — Herpetic eye disease in rabbits after inoculation of autonomic ganglia. *Arch. Ophthal., 97*, 1515, 1979.

Missotten, L. and Maudgal, P.C. — The replica technique used to study superficial corneal epithelium in vivo. *Amer. J. Ophthal., 83*, 104, 1977.

Mitchell, J.E. and McCall, F.C. — Transplacental infection by herpes simplex virus. *Am. J. Dis. Child., 106*, 207, 1963.

Monnet, P. et al. — Meningo-encéphalite herpétique chez un nouveau-né. *Lyon Med., 93*, 209, 1961.

Muller, S.A. — Association of zoster and malignant disorders in children. *Arch. Derm., 96,657*, 1967.

Nahmias, A.J., Alford, C.A. and Korones, S.B. — Infection of the newborn with herpes virus hominis. In: Schulman, I. Ed). Advances in Pediatrics, Vol. 17, Chicago. Year Book Medical Pub. 1970.

Nahmias, A.J., Visintine, A.M., Caldwell, D.R. and Wilson, L.A. — Eye infections with herpes simplex virus in neonates. *Surv. Opthal., 21*, 100, 1976.

Nahmias, A., Visintine, A., Haney, M., Stanwick, T., Lee, F. and Cavanagh, D. — Isolation, quantitation and electron microscopic detection of virus from tears in human herpetic. Relation to antiviral activity. *Adv. Ophthal., 38*, 30, 1979.

Naib, Z., Clepper, A. and Elliott, S. — Exfoliative cytology as an aid in the diagnosis of ophthalmic lesions. *Acta cytol., 11*, 295, 1967.

Nasemann, T. — Pathogenesis of herpes simplex infection of the skin and its relationship to the eye. *Adv. Ophthal., 38*, 24, 1979.

Nauheim, J.S. — Recurrent herpes simplex conjunctival ulceration. *Arch. Ophthal., 81*, 592, 1969.

Neimann, N. et al. — La maladie herpétique du nouveau-né. *Ann. Pediatr., 10*, 27, 1963.

Nesburn, A.B., Elliott, J.H. and Leibowitz, H.M. — Spontaneous reactivation of experimental herpes simplex keratitis in rabbits. *Arch. Ophthal., 78*, 523, 1967.

Nesburn, A.B., Cook, M.L. and Stevens, J.G. — Latent herpes simplex virus. Isolation from rabbit trigeminal ganglia between episodes of recurrent ocular infection. *Arch. Ophthal. 88*, 412, 1972.

Nesburn, A.B., Borit, A., Pentelei-Molnar, J. and Lazaru, R. — Varicella dendritic keratitis. *Invest. Ophthal., 13*, 764, 1974a.

Nesburn, A.B., Robinson, C. and Dickinson, R. — Adenine arabinoside effect on experimental idoxuridine resistant herpes simplex infection. *Invest. Ophthal., 13*, 302, 1974b.

Nesburn, A. B., Dickinson, R., Radnoti, M., and Green, M. J. — Experimental reactivation of ocular herpes simplex in rabbits. *Surv. Ophthal., 21,* 185, 1976a.

Nesburn, A. J., Dickinson, R. and Radnoti, M. — The effect of trigeminal nerve and ganglion manipulation on recurrence of ocular herpes simplex in rabbits. *Invest. Ophthal., 15,* 726, 1976b.

Niedermeier, S. — Behandlung rezidivierender herpetischer Hornhauterkrankungen mit Vidarabin. *Klin. Mbl. Augenheilk., 168,* 713, 1976.

Nowakovsky, S., McGrew, E. A., Medak, H., Burlakow, P. and Nanos, S. — Manifestations of viral infections in exfoliated cells. *Acta Cytol., 12,* 227, 1968.

O'Day, D. M., Poirier, R. H., Jones, D. B. and Elliott, J. H. — Vidarabine therapy of complicated herpes simplex keratitis. *Amer. J. Ophthal., 81,* 642, 1976.

Oh, J. O. and Stevens, T. R. — Comparison of types 1 and 2 herpes virus hominis infection of rabbit eyes: I Clinical manifestations. *Arch. Ophthal., 90,* 473, 1973.

Ormsby, H. L. — Keratoplasty for herpetic keratitis. *Amer. J. Ophthal., 45,* 179, 1958.

Ostler, H. B. — Herpes Simplex: The primary infection. *Surv. Ophthal., 21,* 91, 1976a.

Ostler, H. B. — The management of ocular herpes virus infections. *Surv. Ophthal., 21,* 136, 1976b.

Ostler, H. B. and Thygeson, P. — The ocular manifestations of herpes zoster, varicella, infectious mononucleosis, and cytomegalovirus disease. *Surv. Ophthal., 21,* 148, 1976.

Park, J., Galin, M. A., Billan, A. and Baron, S. — Prophylaxis of herpetic keratoconjunctivitis with interferon inducers. Preliminary observations. *Arch. Ophthal., 81,* 840, 1969.

Partridge, J. W. and Milis, R. R. — Systematic herpes simplex infection in a newborn treated with intravenous idoxuridine. *Arch. Dis. Child., 43,* 377, 1968.

Patterson, A., Fox, A. D., Davies, G. et al. — Controlled studies of IDU in the treatment of herpetic keratitis. *Trans. Ophthal. Soc. U.K., 83,* 589, 1963.

Patterson, A. and Jones, B. R. — The management of ocular herpes. *Trans. Ophthal. Soc. U.K., 87,* 59, 1967.

Pavan-Langston, D. and Nesburn, A. B. — The chronology of primary herpes simplex infection of the eye and adnexal glands. *Arch. Ophthal., 80,* 258, 1968.

Pavan-Langston, D. — New developments in the therapy of ocular herpes simplex. *Int. Ophthal. Clin., 13,* 53, 1973.

Pavan-Langston, D., Dohlman, C. H., Geary, P. A. and Sulzewski, D. — Intraocular penetration of Ara-A and IDU: therapeutic implications in clinical herpetic uveitis. *Trans. Amer. Acad. Ophthal. Otolaryngol., 77,* 455, 1973.

Pavan-Langston, D. and McCulley, J. P. — Herpes zoster dendritic keratitis. *Arch. Ophthal., 89,* 25, 1973.

Pavan-Langston, D., Langston, R. H. S., Geary, P. A. — Prophylaxis and therapy of experimental ocular herpes simplex. Comparison of idoxuridine, adenine arabinoside, and hypoxanthine arabinoside. *Arch. Ophthal., 92,* 417, 1974.

Pavan-Langston, D. — Diagnosis and management of herpes simplex ocular infection. *Int. Ophthal. Clin., 15,* 19, 1975a.

Pavan-Langston, D. — Clinical evaluation of adenine arabinoside and idoxuridine in the treatment of ocular herpes simplex. *Amer. J. Ophthal., 80,* 495, 1975b.

Pavan-Langston, D. and Langston, R. H. S. — Recent advances in antiviral theorapy. *Int. Ophthal. Clinics, 15,* 89, 1975.

Pavan-Langston, D. and Buchanan, R. — Vidarabine therapy of simple and IDU-complicated herpetic keratitis. *Trans. Amer. Acad. Ophthal. Otolaryngol., 81,* OP813, 1976.

Pavan-Langston, D. and Abelson, M. B. — The role of steroids in ocular herpes. In: *Controversy in Ophthalmology.* Bruckhurst, R. J., Boruchoff, S. A., Hutchinson, B. T., Lessell, S. Eds. W. B. Saunders Company, London, 1977.

Pavan-Langston, D. and Foster, C. S. — Trifluorothymidine and idoxuridine therapy of ocular herpes. *Amer. J. Ophthal., 84,* 818, 1977.

Pavan-Langston, D. — Current trends in therapy of ocular herpes simplex: experimental and clinical studies. *Arch. Ophthal., 38,* 82, 1979.

Perkins, E. S., Wood, R. M., Sears, M. L., Prusoff, W. H. and Welch, A. D. — Antiviral activities of several iodinated pyrimidine desoxyribonucleosides. *Nature, 194*, 985, 1962.

Pettay, O. et al. — Herpes simplex virus infection in the newborn. *Arch. Dis. Child., 47,* 97, 1972.

Pettit, T. H., Kimura, S. J. and Peters, H. — Fluorescent antibody technique in diagnosis of herpes simplex keratitis. *Arch. Ophthal., 72,* 86, 1964.

Pfister, R. R., Richards, J. S. F. and Dohlman, C. H. — Recurrence of herpetic keratitis in corneal grafts. *Amer. J. Ophthal., 73,* 192, 1972.

Piebenga, L. W. and Laibson, P. R. — Dendritic lesions in herpes zoster ophthalmicus. *Arch. Ophthal., 90,* 268, 1973.

Pierce, L. E. and Jenkins, R. B. — Herpes zoster ophthalmicus treated with cytarabine. *Arch. Ophthal., 89,* 21, 1973.

Pillard, R., Wildi, E. and Wirth, J. — Herpes simplex du nouveau-né (complications encéphalitique; mise en évidence expérimentale de l'agent causal). *Dermatologica, 100,* 285, 1950.

Plotkin, J., Reynaud, A, and Okumoto, M. — Cytologic study of herpetic keratitis. *Arch. Ophthal., 85,* 597, 1971.

Polack, E. M. and Kaufman, H. E. — Penetrating keratoplasty in herpetic keratitis. *Amer. J. Ophthal., 73,* 908, 1972.

Private de Garhile, M. and De Rudder. J. — Effet de deux nucléoside de l'arabinose sur la multiplication des virus de l'herpès et de la vaccine en culture cellulaire. *C.R. Acad. Sci., 259,* 2725, 1964.

Proto, F. and Tedesco, N. — Observazioni su di un coso di cheratite erpetica neonatale. *Boll. Oculist., 45,* 573, 1966.

Prusoff, W. H., Chen, M. S., Fischer, P. H., Lin, T. S., Shiau, G. T. and Schinazi, R. F. — Role of nucleosides in virus and cancer chemotherapy. *Adv. Ophthal., 38,* 3, 1979.

Quéré, M. A., Diallo, J. and Rogez, J. P. La Kératite de Thygeson (a propos de 16 cas de Kératite pontuée superficielle). *Bull. Soc. Ophthal. Fr., 67,* 276, 1967.

Quilligan, J. J. Jr. and Wilson, J. L. — Fatal herpes simplex infection in a newborn infant. *J. Lab. and Chin. Med., 38,* 742, 1951.

Rapp, F. and Vanderslice, D. — Spread of zoster virus in human empryonic lung cells and the inhibitory effect of iododeoxy-uridine. *Virology, 22,* 321, 1964.

Ribble, J. C. — Chickenpox (varicella). In: *Harrison's Principles of Internal Medicine.* Wintrobe et al. (eds.) McGraw Hill Book Company. New York, 1970, p. 993.

Rice, N. S. C. and Jones, B. R. — Problems of corneal grafting in herpetic keratitis. In: *Ciba Foundation Symposium on Corneal Graft Failure.* Associated Scientific Publishers, London, Vol. 15, 1973.

Richards, A. B., Bowbyes, J. and Jones, B. R. — Cryotherapy of epithelial herpes simplex keratitis. *Amer. J. Ophthal., 73,* 45, 1977.

Rogers, W., Hartman, A., Palm, P., Okstein, C. and Kensler, C. — The fate of 5-trifluoromethyl-2'-deoxyuridine in monkeys, dogs, mice and tumor-bearing mice. *Cancer Res., 29,* 953, 1969.

Ross, J. V. M. — Herpes zoster ophthalmicus sine eruption. *Arch. Ophthal., 42,* 808, 1949.

Schabel, F. M., Jr. — The antiviral activity of 9-β-D-arabinofuranosyladenine (Ara-A). *Chemotherapy, 13,* 321, 1968.

Schanbrum, E., Miller, S. and Haar, H. — Herpes zoster in hematologic neoplasias: some unusual manifestations. *Ann. Int. Med., 53,* 522, 1960.

Scheie, H. — Treatment of herpes zoster ophthalmicus with cortisone or corticotropin. *Arch. Ophthal., 53,* 38, 1955.

Scheie, H. and McLellan, T. — Treatment of herpes zoster ophthalmicus with corticotropin and corticosteroids. *Arch. Ophthal., 62,* 579, 1959.

Schwartz, J. and Roizman, B. — Concerning the egress of herpes simplex virus form infected cells: Electron and light microscope observations. *Virology, 38,* 42, 1969.

Schweitzer, N. M. J. — A fluorescein colored polygonal pattern in the human cornea, the reflectographic "Furchenbild" of Fischer. *Arch. Ophthal.,* 548, 1967.

Scott, T. F. M. — Epidemiology of herpetic infections. *Amer. J. Ophthal., 43,* 134, 1957.

Scriba, M. — Herpes simplex virus infection in guinnae pigs: an animal model for studying latent and recurrent herpes simplex virus infection. *Infect. Immun., 12,* 162, 1975.

Sidwell, R.W., Arnett, G. and Dixon, G.L. — Effect of selected biologically active compounds on in vitro cytomegalovirus (CMV) infections. Abstracts of papers. *7th Intersci. Conf. Antimicr. Agents and Chemotherapy.* Abs. no. 64, pp. 28-29, 1967.

Sidwell, R.W., Dixon, G.J., Sellers, S.M. and Schabel, F.M.Jr. — In vivo antiviral properties of biologically active compounds II. Studies with influenza and vaccinia viruses. *Appl. Microbiol., 16,* 370, 1968a.

Sidwell, R.W., Dixon, G.J., Schabel, Jr. F.M. and Kaump, D.H. — Antiviral activity of 9-β-D-arabinofuranosyladenine II. Activity against herpes simplex keratitis in hamsters. *Antimicrob. Agents Chemother., 8,* 148, 1968b.

Sidwell, R.W., Allen, L.B., Huffman, J.H. et al. — Viral keratitis inhibitory effect of 9-β-D-arabinofuranosylhypoxanthine 5'-monophosphate. *Antimicrob. Agents Chemother., 8,* 463, 1975.

Singha, S.S. and Nirankari, M.S. — Herpes zoster ophthalmicus. *Orient. Arch. Ophthal., 8,* 21, 1970.

Sloan, B.J. — Adenine arabinoside chemotherapy studies in animals. In: *Adenine Arabinoside: An antiviral agent.* Pavan-Langston, D., Buchanan, R.A and Alford, Jr. C.A., New York, Raven Press 1975.

Smith, M.G., Lennette, E.H. and Reames, H.R. — Isolation of the virus of herpes simplex and the demonstration of intranuclear inclusions in a case of acute encephalitis. *Amer. J. Pathol., 17,* 55, 1941.

Smith, I.W., Peutherer, J.F. and MacCallum, F.O. — The incidence of Herpesvirus hominis antibody in the populaι ιι. *J. Hyg., 65,* 395, 1967.

Sokal, J.E. and Firat, D. — Varicella-zoster infection in Hodgkin's disease. *Amer. J. Med., 39,* 452, 1965.

Soltz-Szots, J. — Zur serologie des Herpes simplex. *Arch. Klin. Exp. Derm., 209,* 121, 1959.

Sood, N.N. and Marmion, V.J. — Superficial herpetic keratitis treated with 5-iodo-2'-deoxyuridine. *Brit. J. Ophthal., 48,* 609, 1964.

Spinak, M. — Cytology as an aid in the study of ocular diseases. In: *XXIII concilium diagnosticum Acta.* Pars II; Kyoto, 1978, Excerpta Medica, Amsterdam, 1979.

Stevens, J.G. and Cook, M.L. — Latent herpes simplex virus in spinal ganglia of mice. *Science, 173,* 843, 1971.

Stevens, J.G., Nesburn, A.B. and Cook, M.L. — Latent herpes simplex virus from trigeminal ganglia of rabbits with recurrent eye infection. *Nature, 235,* 216, 1972.

Stevens, J.G. and Cook, M.L. — Maintenance of latent herpetic infection: an apparent role for antiviral IgG. *J. Immunol., 113,* 1685, 1974.

Sugar, J., Varnell, E., Centifanto, Y. and Kaufman, H.E. — Trifluorothymidine treatment of herpetic iritis in rabbits and ocular penetration. *Invest. Ophthal., 12,* 532, 1973.

Sugar, H.S. — Herpetic Keratouveitis, Clinical experiences. *Ann. Ophthal. 3,* 355, 1971.

Sugiura, S. and Kondo. E. — Development of dendritic keratitis on the cornea of the rabbit after previous resection of the trigeminal nerve. *Acta Soc. Ophthal. Jap., 65,* 502, 1961.

Sugiura, S. and Wakui, K. — Polygonal cell at the basal cell layer of the corneal epithelium of man with special reference to its role in movement of the ocular fluids. *Acta Soc. Ophthal. Jap., 65,* 2434, 1961.

Sugiura, S. and Kondo, E. — Development of dendritic keratitis on the corneal graft of the rabbit. Study on the morphogenesis of dendritic keratitis. *Acta. Soc. Ophthal. Jap., 66,* 13, 1962.

Sundmacher, R., Neumann-Haefelin, D. and Cantell, K. — Successful treatment of dendritic keratitis with human leukocyte interferon. *Alb. v. Graefes Arch. Klin. Exp. Ophthal., 201,* 39, 1976.

Sundmacher, R., Cantell, K., Skoda, R. et al. — Human leukocyte and fibroblast interferon in a combination therapy of dendritic keratitis. *Alb. v. Graefes Arch. Klin. Exp. Ophthal., 208,* 229, 1978.

Takahashi, G. H., Leibowitz, H. M. and Kibrick, S. — Topically applied steroids in active herpes simplex keratitis. *Arch. Ophthal., 85,* 350, 1971.

Takemura, T. — Electron microscope study of human herpetic keratitis (on the tenth day after the onset of typical dendritic keratitis). *Exp. Eye Res., 2,* 305, 1963.

Takemura, T. and Kitano, S. — Studies on herpes corneae: III electron microscopic observation on the experimental herpetic keratitis in rabbits (findings on 18 hrs and 52 hrs after inoculation of herpes simplex virus). *Acta Soc. Ophthal. Jap., 64,* 2979, 1960.

Tamm, I. — Symposium on the experimental pharmacology and clinical use of antimetabolites: III Metabolic antagonist and selective virus inhibition. *Clin. Pharmacol. Ther., 1,* 777, 1960.

Tanaka, N. and Kimura, S. J. — Localization of herpes simplex antigen and virus: In the corneal stroma of experimental herpetic keratitis. *Arch. Ophthal., 78,* 68, 1967.

Tanaka, N. and Togni, B. — Further investigations by electron microscopy of herpes simplex virus in the corneal stroma of rabbits with experimental keratitis. *Exp. Eye Res., 7,* 142, 1968.

Tarakji, M. S., Matta, C. S. and Shammaj, H. F. — Cryotherapy of herpes simplex keratitis. *Ann. Ophthal., 10,* 1557, 1978.

Thygeson, P. — Cytologic observations on herpetic keratitis. *Amer, J. Ophthal., 45,* 240, 1958.

Thygeson, P. — Ocular viral diseases. *Med. Clin. N. Amer., 43,* 1419, 1959.

Thygeson, P. — Marginal herpes simplex keratitis simulating catarrhal ulcer. *Invest. Ophthal., 10,* 1006, 1971.

Thygeson, P. — The unfavorable role of corticosteroids in herpetic keratitis. In: *controversery in ophthalmology.* Brockhurst, R. J., Boruchoff, S, A., Hutchinson, B. T., Lessel, S. Eds. W. B. Saunders Company, London, 1977.

Tokumaru, T. — Production of epinephrine-induced skin lesions and fever following local and systemic injections of herpes simplex and vascular stomatitis viruses in the rabbit. *Arch. Ges. Virusforsch., 34,* 179, 1971.

Tomasi, T. B. Jr. — Human immunoglobulin A. *N. Engl. J. Med., 279,* 1327, 1968.

Trobe, J. D., Centifanto, Y., Zam, Z. S. et al. — Anti-herpes activity of adenine arabinoside monophosphate. *Invest. Ophthal., 15,* 196, 1976.

Uchida, Y. and Kimura, S. J. — Fluorescent antibody localization of herpes simplex virus in the conjunctiva. *Arch. Ophthal., 73,* 413, 1965.

Uchida, Y., Kameyama, K. and Kaneko, M. — Etiological diagnosis of herpetic keratitis. *Jap. J. Ophthal., 16,* 3, 1974.

Vidal, J. B. — Inoculabilité des pustules d'ecthyma. *Ann. Dermatol. Syph. (Paris), 4,* 350, 1873.

Van Horn, D. L., Edelhauser, H. F. and Schultz, R. O. — Experimental herpes simplex keratitis. Early alterations of corneal epithelium and stroma. *Arch. Ophthal., 84,* 67, 1970.

Walsh, F. B. and Hoyt, W. F. — Clinical neuro-ophthalmology. Williams and Wilkins Co. Baltimore, 1969, p. 1355.

Walz, M. A., Price, R. W. and Notkins, A. L. — Latent infection with herpes simplex virus type 1 and 2. Viral reactivation in vivo after neurectomy. *Science, 184,* 1185, 1974.

Watson, D. H. — Morphology. In: Kaplan, A. S. (Ed.). The herpes viruses. Academic Press, New York, 1973.

Weddell, G. and Zander, E. — A critical evaluation of methods used to demonstrate tissue ocular elements illustrated by reference to the cornea. *J. Anat. (London), 84,* 168, 1950.

Weissenbacher, M., Galin, M. A., Chowchuvech, E. et al. — Protection by polynosinic-polycytidilic acid complex of rabbit eye tissue cultures infected with herpes simplex virus. Effect of neomycin and virus challange dose. *Invest. Ophthal., 9,* 857, 1970.

Wellings, T., Awdry, P., Bors, F., Jones, B. R., Brown, D. and Kaufman, H. E. — Clinical evaluation of trifluorothymidine in the treatment of herpes simplex corneal ulcers. *Amer. J. Ophthal., 79,* 932, 1972.

Wheeler, C.E., Jr. — Kaposis Varicelliform eruption. In: Dennis, D.J., Crounse, R.G., Dobson, R.L. and McGuire, J. (eds): *Clinical dermatology.* Vol. 3, Hagerstown, M.D. Harper and Row, 1973.

Whitcher, J.P., Dawson, C.R., Hoshiwara, I., Daghpous, T., Messadi, M., Triki, F. and Oh, J.O. — Herpes simplex keratitis in a developing country. Natural history and treatment of epithelial ulcers in Tunisia. *Arch. Ophthal., 94,* 587, 1976.

Whitman, L., Wall, M.J. and Warren, J. — Herpes simplex encephalitis. A report of two fatal cases. *J.A.M.A., 131,* 1408, 1946.

Wildy, P. — The progression of herpes simplex virus to the central nervous system of the mouse. *J. Hyg., 65,* 173, 1967.

Wildy, P. — Herpes: History and classification. In: Kaplan, A.S. (Ed.) The herpes viruses. Academic Press, New York, 1973.

Yamaguchi, K., Okumoto, M., Stern, G., Friedlaender, M. and Smolin, G. — Idoxuridine and bacterial corneal infection. *Amer. J. Ophthal., 87,* 202, 1979.

Yen, S., Reagen, J. and Rosenthal, M. — Herpes simplex infection in female genital tract. *Obstet. Gynecol., 25,* 479, 1965.

Zarafonetis, C.J.D., Smadel, J.E., Adams, J.W. and Haymaker, W. — Fatal herpes simplex encephalitis in man. *Amer. J. Path., 201,* 429, 1944.

Zuelzer, W.W. and Stulberg, C.S. — Herpes simplex virus as a cause of fulminating visceral disease and hepatitis in infancy: Report of eight cases and isolation of virus in one case. *Amer. J. Dis. Child., 83,* 421, 1952.

CHAPTER IX

THE DRY EYE SYNDROME

A dry eye may be defined as the eye which exhibits an abnormal corneal epithelium secondary to an abnormal precorneal tear film (Baum, 1976). Such a broad clinical definition includes the etiological factors of tear film abnormalities due to deficiency of tear film composition, the corneal and conjunctival surface abnormalities, and the mechanical factors which may not allow proper dispersion of tear film on the cornea. In the last two conditions there is generally adequate tear secretion. The common essential feature is, however, an area of corneal dry surface.

A detailed discussion of all the etiological conditions (Table IX-1) is beyond the scope of this report. The clinical picture of dry cornea due to surface abnormalities and defective spreading of tear film can be easily recognised on the basis of associated etiological conditions. On the contrary tear deficiency conditions give rise to typical corneal appearance, irrespective of underlying cause. In this category kerato-conjunctivitis sicca is a frequent condition resulting from a serious lack of tear secretion in Sjögren's syndrome. Deficiencies of the mucus or lipid components generally produce dry spots on the cornea.

TABLE I. — *Dry eye: etiological conditions*

I. Alterations in the tear film composition.

   A. Aqueous deficiency:

      a. *Congenital:*
        1. aplasia or hypoplasia of the lacrimal gland (alacrimia congenita, Bonne-ville-Ullrich syndrome)
        2. anhydrotic ectodermal dysplasia
        3. aplasia of lacrimal nerve nucleus
        4. congenital familial sensory neuropathy with anhydrosis
        5. familial autonomic dysfunction (Riley-Day Syndrome)
        6. Holmes-Adie syndrome (Pupillotonia, hyporeflexia, segmental hypohy-drosis)
        7. multiple endocrine neoplasia

TABLE I. *(continued)*

b. *Acquired:*
1. senile atrophy of lacrimal gland
2. idiopathic atrophy of lacrimal gland
3. atropy or hypofunction of the lacrimal gland associated with systemic diseases:
    a) connective tissue diseases
        rheumatoid arthritis
        systemic lupus erythematosis
        periarteritis nodosa
        scleroderma
    b) hematopoietic and reticulo–endothelial disorders
        Felty's syndrome
        malignant lymphoma
        lymphosarcoma
        thrombocytopenic purpura
        lymphoid leukaemia
        hemolytic anemia
        hypergammaglobulinemia
        Waldenström's macroglobulinemia
        chronic hepatitis
        cirrhosis of liver
    c) endocrine dysfunction
        Hashimotos disease
        climacteric in females
    d) renal disorders:
        renal tubular acidosis
        diabetes inspidus
    e) skin and mucocutaneous diseases (mainly cause mucus deficiency but may reduce aqueous tear flow due to scar formation)
        psoriasis arthropathica
        acanthosis nigricans
        scleroderma
        erythema multiforme (Stevens Jonhnson's syndrome)
        exfoliative dermatitis
        ocular pemphigoid
        dermatitis herptiformis
        epidermolysis bullosa
        ichthyosiform erytheroderma
        acne rosacea
        congenital ichthyósis
    f) miscellaneous
        sarcoidosis
        adult coeliac disease
        amyloidosis
        lipodystropy
        late-life myopathy
4. post surgical:
    partial or total dacryoadenectomies
    after blepharoplasty
5. traumatic, inflammatory or neoplastic lesions of the lacrimal gland
6. neuroparalytic:
    lesions of VII nerve and geniculate ganglion
    lesions of greater superficial petrosal nerve
    lesions of sphenopalatine ganglion and the lacrimal branch
    lesions of trigeminal nerve, including Gasserian ganglion

TABLE I *(continued)*

7. toxic and iatrogenic
    belladona and its alkaloids
    botulism
    deep anaesthesia
    practalol
8. nutritional and debilitating disorders
    typhus
    cholera
    high fever
    starvation
    ascorbic acid and Vit. B_{12} deficiency (?)

B. Mucus deficiency:
    vitamine A deficiency
    Reiter's disease
    diphtheric keratoconjunctivitis
    trachoma
    includes the mucocutaneous disorders enumerated above
    chemical, thermal and radiational injuries of the conjunctiva
    iatrogenic: echothiophate iodide (phospholine iodide), sulfonamides and practalol

C. Lipid deficiency: chronic blepharitis

II. Surface abnormalities causing faulty tear-film dispersion:

A. Focal elevations on corneal surface:
    multiple forms of punctate epithelial keratitis
    Salzman's nodular dystrophy
    phlyctenule formation
    waxy corneal ulcer

B. Elevations at limbus leading to dellen formation:
    pterygium
    pinguecula
    postoperative inflammatory reaction

C. Improper contact lens wear.

III. Defective spreading of the tear film:

a. alterations of blink mechanism
    CNS disorders
    hyperthyroidism
    drug induced
    after contact lens wear
b. lagophthalmos
    facial palsy
    nocturnal lagophthalmos
    scars of the lids
c. mechanical factors
    exophthalmos
    ectropion
    symblepharon

Modified after Maudgal, 1976; Jones 1977 and Ruprecht et al., 1977.

DRY SPOTS

Marx (1921) described "dry spot" as a dark hole developing in the fluorescein-stained precorneal tearfilm a short time after a complete blink. Dry spots are a pathological finding if they develop in less than 10 seconds after blinking. (Lemp et al., 1971). In normal eyes dry spots or lines in the tear film appear in 15 to 40 seconds if the lids are kept apart after a blink. (Norn, 1969; Dohlman et al., 1970).

Etiology

Dry spots may develop due to an alteration in the epithelium or tear film. They are commonly seen in the superficial epithelial diseases of the cornea. The altered epithelial cells project from the corneal surface producing localized alterations in the precorneal tear film. In these cases there may not be any quantitative or qualitative abnormalities of the precorneal film. Dry spots are more frequently seen in keratoconjunctivitis sicca (Brown, 1970). Since mucoid and lipid layers of the tear film play an important role in the spread and stabilization of the precorneal film, their deficient secretion may result in dry spots on the cornea even in the presence of adequate aqueous secretion. (Lemp et al., 1970a, 1970b, 1971; Holly and Lemp, 1971a; Holly, 1973).

Pathology

Repeated appearance of dry spots may lead to localized areas of epithelial dehydration resulting in cellular damage which in turn disrupts the tear film and starts a vicious circle. In experimental studies (Pfister and Renner, 1977) epithelium cells in the areas of dry spots show loss of surface microvilli, plasmalemmal disintegration and exfoliation. In small spots as few as 5 superficial cells were involved but the larger ones were characterised by epithelial defects involving loss of two or three layers of cells. Similar but more extensive cellular damage has been shown to occur if the rabbit eyes are kept open for 30 minutes at room temperature (Brewitt and Bonatz, 1979).

Clinical picture

Our patients in whom dry spots on the cornea were detected, complained of mild irritation and pricking sensation at irregular intervals; relieved by frequent blinking. In most cases the eyes were white but in severe cases in whom numerous dry spots developed rapidly, the bulbar conjunctiva showed slight to moderate injection.

On examination the tear-film breaks up immediately after a blink and if the eye is prevented from blinking, epithelial alterations begin to appear within a few seconds. The epithelial dry spots are best seen in retro illumination and can actually be observed enlarging during examination . They are transparent lesions with irregular surface, varying in form from irregular spots to stellate pseudo- dendritic figures (figs. IX-1 and IX-2). They may change their shape and

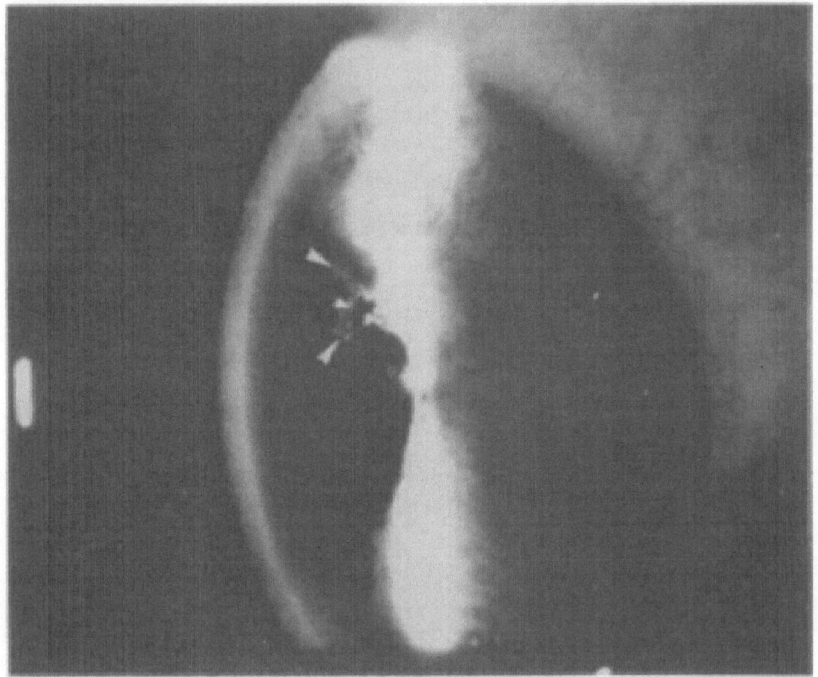

Fig. IX-1. — Epithelial dry spot (arrows) on the cornea.

appear at different sites on different examinations. However, if advanced epithelial changes have occured they may remain localized to a particular area. The epithelial lesions disappear if the patient is

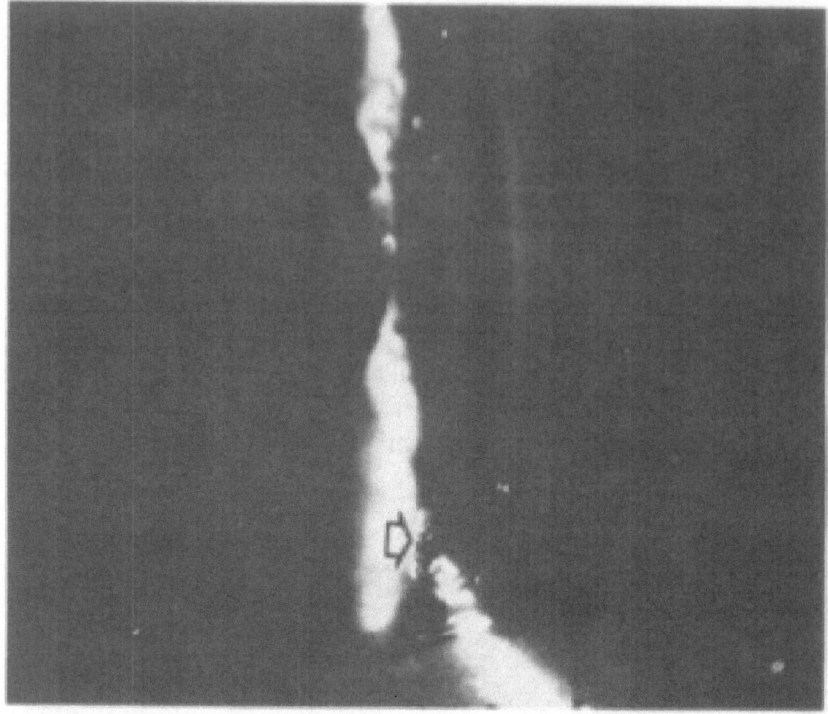

Fig. IX-2. — Dendritic-form dry spot (arrows) on the cornea.

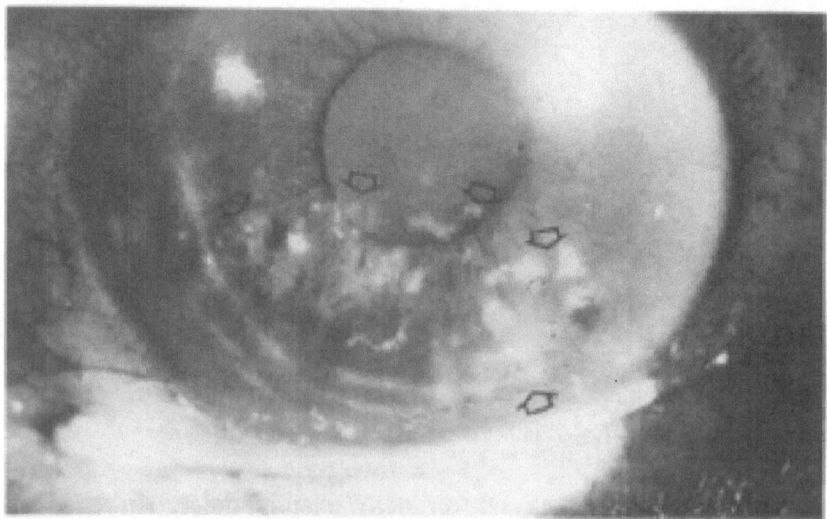

Fig. IX-3. — Multiple fluorescein stained dry spots (some indicated by arrows) in a patient with zero BUT.

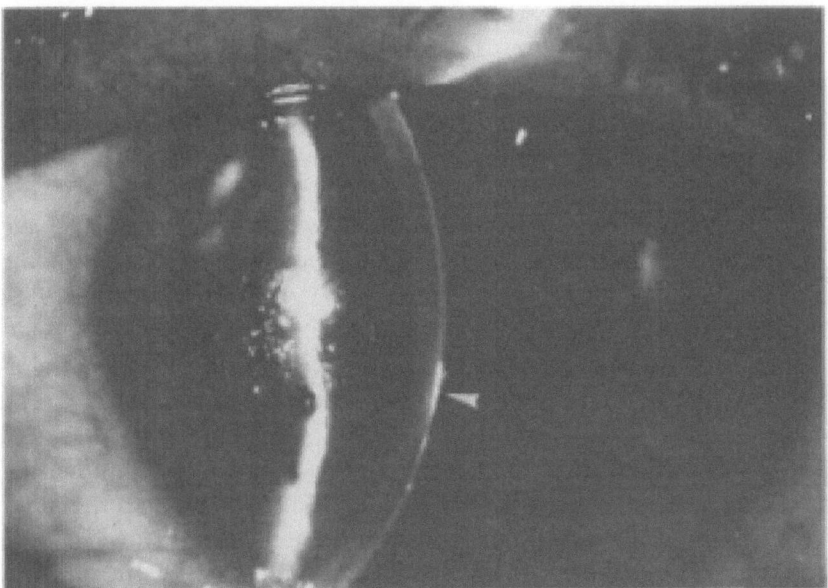

Fig. IX-4. — Slit-beam photograph of the dry spots shown in figure IX-3. The lesions are limited to the epithelium (arrow).

asked to blink a few times rapidly or if the eyes are kept closed for a few seconds. But in patients with zero break-up time new lesions appear quickly even between normal blinks (figs. IX-3 and IX-4). Fluorescein stains the affected area of the epithelium if instilled after the lesions have appeared and before the next blink. If one is looking for dry spots in a fluorescein stained tearfilm the newly developing epithelial lesions may remain unstained.

In a severe form dry spots may lead to epithelial erosions or dellen formation. (Baum et al., 1968; Brown, 1973; Pfister and Renner, 1977).

Treatment of dry spots is discussed under the therapy of dry eye conditions.

KERATOCONJUNCTIVITIS SICCA (KCS)

It is a major component of Sjögren's syndrome (Sjögren, 1933) which is primarily a chronic benign disorder of obscure etiology. Accompanying features are xerostomia (dry mouth) and rheumatoid arthritis or connective tissue diseases.

Sjögren's syndrome

Apart from ocular symptoms, polyarthritis and decreased salivary secretions, secretory glands of the body may be affected involving nasophryngeal, buccal, oesophageal, tracheo-broncheal, genital and sweat glands alongwith the symptoms of collagen disease. Since Hendrik Sjögren's monograph (1933) there have been considerable reports in literature showing the widespread systemic nature of the affection (Appelmans, 1948; Henderson, 1950; Coverdale, 1955; McLenachan, 1956; Ramage and Kinnear, 1956; Paczesniak, 1957; Gamp, 1958; Kologlu, 1958; Denko and Bergenstal, 1960; Ferreira-Marques, 1960; Bertram et al., 1961; Vanselow et al., 1963; Crews and Whitfield, 1963; Bunim et al., 1964; Nagakura and Nagakura, 1964; Pangrati, 1964; Bloch et al., 1965; Flynn and Schulmeister, 1967; Escande and Degos, 1968; Sood, 1968; and many others).

Most of the patients are females past menopause. However, the condition may develop at any adult age and has been reported in males. The ocular symptoms may precede or follow the onset of rheumatoid arthritis and there may be a considerable interval between the two. Sjögren's syndrome is rare in children. O'Neil (1965) reported its development in a 10 year old girl and Radnot & Wallner (1954) in a child of 6 years age.

The patient may complain of dryness of mouth, nose, pharynx and oesophagus leading to fissured mouth and tongue; difficulty in mastication and swallowing; crust formation in the nose and chronic cough. Dryness of the genital passages and decreased sweating may cause pruritis ani and vulvae. Some cases show loss of body hair. Recurrent episodes of parotid or other salivary gland enlargement may be present or may have occurred in the past. There may not be any history of lacrimal gland enlargement. Some patients may show associated thyroid gland involvement.

In addition to general weakness and fatigue, features of achylia gastrica, hypochromic anaemia, hepatomegaly, splenomegaly, vascular disorders and dental caries have been reported. The commonest systemic association in Sjögren's syndrome is rheumatoid arthritis which is clinically and radiologically indistinguishable from arthritis without sicca symptoms. In the series of Bloch et al. (1965) 87% of the patients had rheumatoid arthritis.

Sjögren's syndrome has been reported with other connective tissue diseases (Bloch and Bunim 1963); SLE (Heaton, 1959; Horan, 1969;

Bowers, 1969; Steinberg and Talal, 1971); Scleroderma (Escande and Degos, 1968; Kirkham, 1969); polyarteritis nodosa (Stanworth, 1951; Ramage and Kinnear, 1956; Hardsky et al., 1968). Raynaud's phenomenon may occur in these patients (Bloch et al., 1965; Guilaine et al., 1970). Fox (1966) reported a case with late-life myopathy.

An association with lymphoid leukaemia (Jézégabel et al., 1966; Lehner-Netsch et al., 1969; Heindle, 1967); lymphosarcoma and malignant lymphoma (Talal and Bunim, 1964), lymphoreticulosarcoma (Haye et al., 1968) nodular reticulum cell sarcoma (Hornbaker et al., 1966) thyroid disease (Stoltze et al., 1960; Remolar et al., 1965; Walser et al., 1965) has been reported.

Steinberg et al. (1971) described three cases in which fatal thrombotic thrombocytopenic purpura developed. Fogel (1959) reported a case of benign purpura. Haemolytic anaemia (Bowers, 1969; Lehner-Netsch et al., 1969), Felty's Syndrome (Rozenblit and Tenezynska, 1965), hypergammaglobulinaemia (Fogel, 1959; Stoltze et al., 1960; Bunim, 1965), primary amyloidosis (Kuczynski et al., 1971), adult coeliac disease (Pittman and Holub, 1965), renal tubular acidosis (Shioji et al., 1970), nephrogenic diabetes insipidus (Shearn and Tu, 1965), Bernier-Boek's disease (De Haas, 1952), have also been documented with Sjögren's syndrome.

Hood et al. (1970) reported the development of Sjögren's syndrome on deprivation of ascorbic acid which was ameliorated by ascorbic acid treatment. Kuming and Politzer (1967) described association of protein malnutrition with Sjögren's syndrome in Bantu children, and Wegelius et al. (1970) and Williamson et al. (1970) reported Vitamin B_{12} deficiency due to the presence of antibodies to the gastric parietal cells and Addisonian pernicious anaemia.

Occurrence of benign lympho-epithelial lesions of the lacrimal gland have been found in 40% of the patients suffering from Sjögren's syndrome (Vanselow et al., 1963; Bloch et al., 1965).

Etiology

In recent years, the involvement of auto-immune mechanisms in Sjögren's syndrome has been stressed. The presence of anti-nuclear auto-antibodies (Bloch et al., 1965; Beck et al., 1965; Guilaine et al., 1970) and antibodies directed against salivary glands or their duct cells have been reported (Anderson et al., 1961; Denko, 1965; Feltkamp and Van Rossum, 1968). In their in vivo experiments, Leventhal and associates (1967), demonstrated development of delayed hypersensitivity to 2,4-dinitrochlorobenzene skin sensitization and in vitro impaired lymphocyte transformation in patients with Sjögren's syndrome. Autoimmune liver disease may also be associated with keratitis sicca (McFarlane et al., 1976).

The histopathology of the lacrimal and salivary glands has been studied by many workers. There is atrophy of the acini with round cell infiltration. Progressive connective tissue proliferation occurs which replaces most of the secretory parenchyma in advanced cases. Eventually fibrosis follows. Similar changes may occur in the accessory glands of Krause, mucus glands of lips and larynx. Hyaline and cystic degeneration may be seen in fibrotic areas.

Bloch et al. (1965) reported atrophy of the submucus glands with lymphocytic infiltration of the respiratory tract and pulmonary complications i.e. pneumonia, atelectasis and fibrosis.

Ocular involvement

Keratoconjunctivitis sicca (KCS) was the term first used by Sjögren (1933) to describe the pathological condition of dry eye and the typical picture resulting from it. Duke-Elder (1965) defined it as "chronic intractable, irritable conjunctivitis unrelieved by treatment, characterised by a ropy mucoid discharge and often associated with epithelial roughening and the development of fine corneal erosions and filamentary keratitis".

Clinical picture

This disease is of gradual onset, usually bilateral but may be more pronounced on one side. The patient may complain of burning, smarting, roughness, grittiness or a foreign body sensation in the eye, accompanied by mild redness of the conjunctiva and thick ropy discharge which is variously described as tenacious or thready, yellowish, mucoid discharge (fig. IX-5). Some patients complain of swelling of the eyes in the morning which improves as the day progresses.

On *biomicroscopy* there may be much less to see in relation to what the patient complains. There is mild conjunctival injection with rough lusterless corneal surface staining with rose bengal or fluorescein solutions (fig. IX-6). Sometimes epithelial filaments form. Asso-

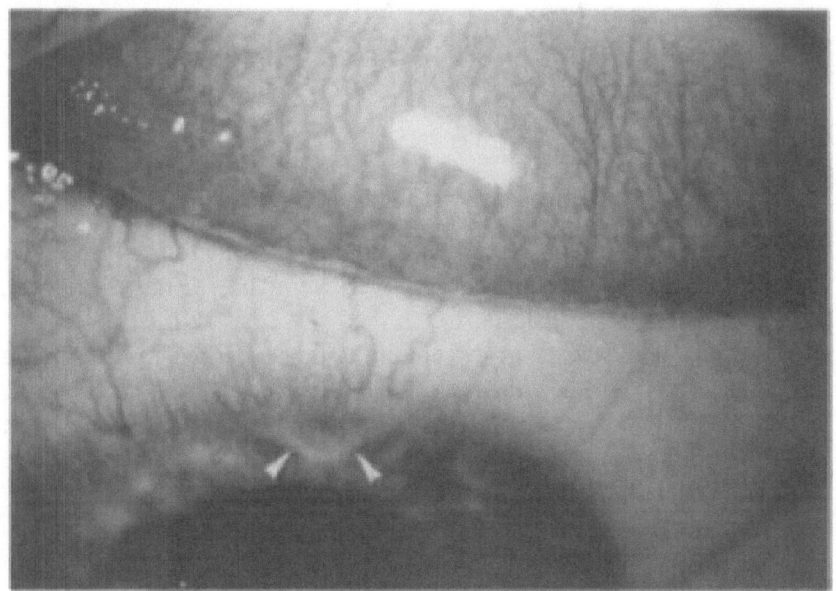

Fig. IX-5. — Thready mucoid secretion in KCS.

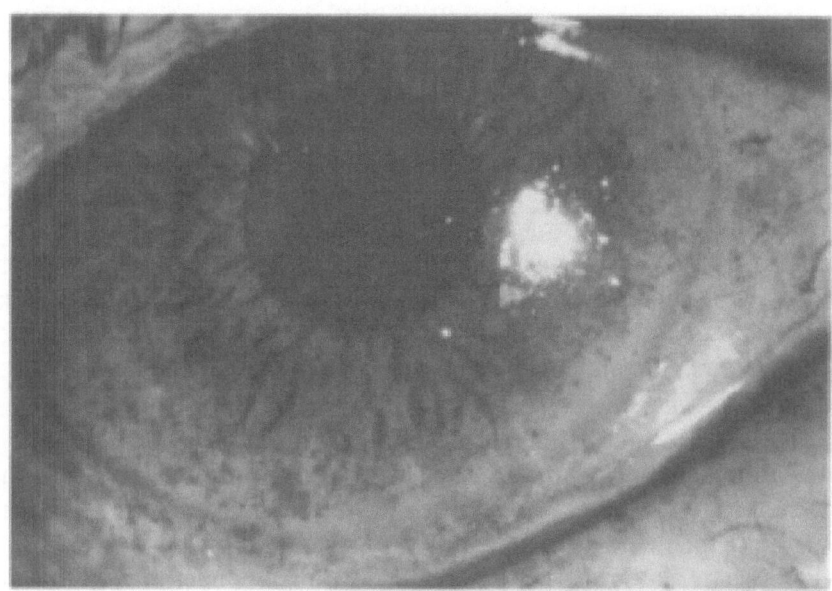

Fig. IX-6. — Rose bengal punctate staining of the cornea in KCS.

ciated infection, mostly by staphylococci (Williamson et al., 1971, Maudgal, 1976), may be present.

Pathogenesis and Pathology

The corneal epithelium becomes initially edematous if the tear secreting glands of rabbit are removed surgically (François et al., 1974 and 1976; Maudgal, 1976).

Histopathology shows that the edema is most marked in the middle layers where hydropic degeneration may occur. The edematous response, however, does not remain uniform. Hydropic degeneration leads to thinning of the epithelium in some parts of the cornea while at other places hypertrophy may ensue.

In the area of hypertrophy the cells of middle layer have a tendency of "rosette" arrangment. Occasionally a patch of epithelium may become markedly hypertropic which appears spindle shaped in transverse sections. At the same time keratohyalin begins to form in the basal layers of cells, which gradually progresses to electron dense intracellular filaments of keratin as the cell migrates to the corneal surface (François et al., 1976; Maudgal, 1976). Multilayered keratinised cells form a lamellar pattern on the surfaces of the cornea, but their desmosomal attachments are broken, the nuclei are fragmented and the surface plasma membranes may rupture, so that the keratinised filaments extrude from the cells. The keratinised surface cells, however, still possess some DNA and RNA, unlike the keratinised cells of skin, nails, hoof and hair (Maudgal and Missotten, 1978). Also the superficial keratinised cells are smaller and irregularly arranged than the normal surface epithelium cells. Some cells are detached and others appear piled up on each other (figs. IX-7 and IX-8). On scanning electron microscopy, the keratinised cells appear dark due to the loss of microvilli and are devoid of surface craters. The basement membrane is thinned and irregular (Maudgal, 1976). There are a large number of Teng cells.

The conjunctival epithelium is similarly keratinised. Goblet cells are atrophic, few in numbers and displaced towards the surface. In some areas they are totally absent. The submucosal elastic tissue becomes fragmented (Maudgal, 1976).

Corneal filament formation occurs by migration of the epithelial cells around the focal areas of cell necrosis (see Chapter V).

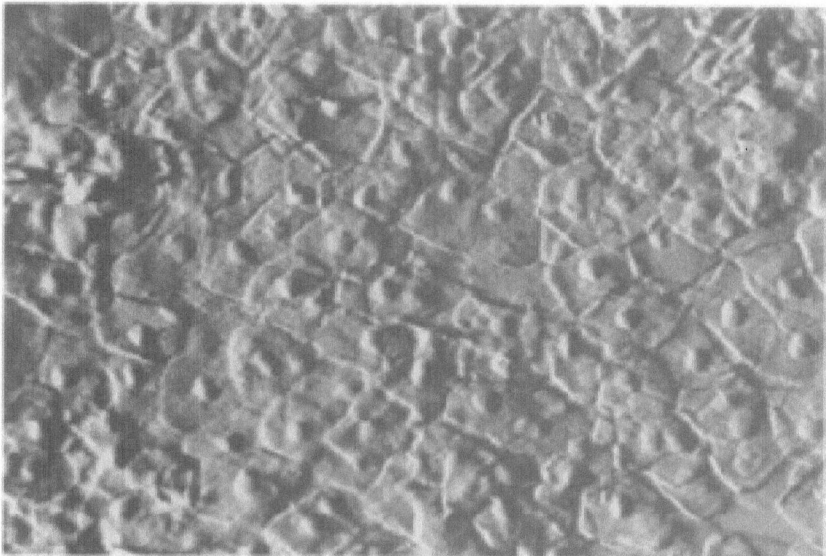

Fig. IX-7. — Experimental KCS showing irregularly arranged, piled up or partly detached superficial keratinised cells of the epithelium. Corneal replica technique. Oblique illumination microscopy. × 160.

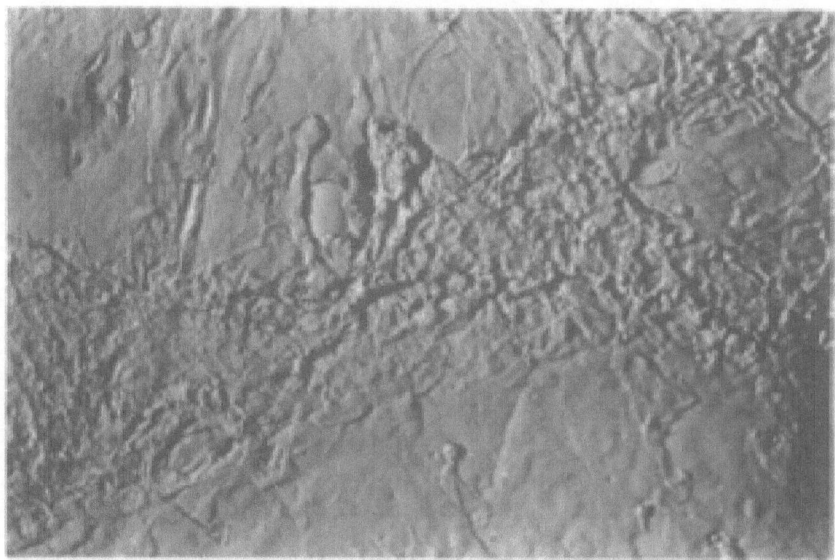

Fig. IX-8. — Flat mount of superficial epithelium in experimental KCS showing a degenerated cell (arrow). Corneal replica technique. × 410.

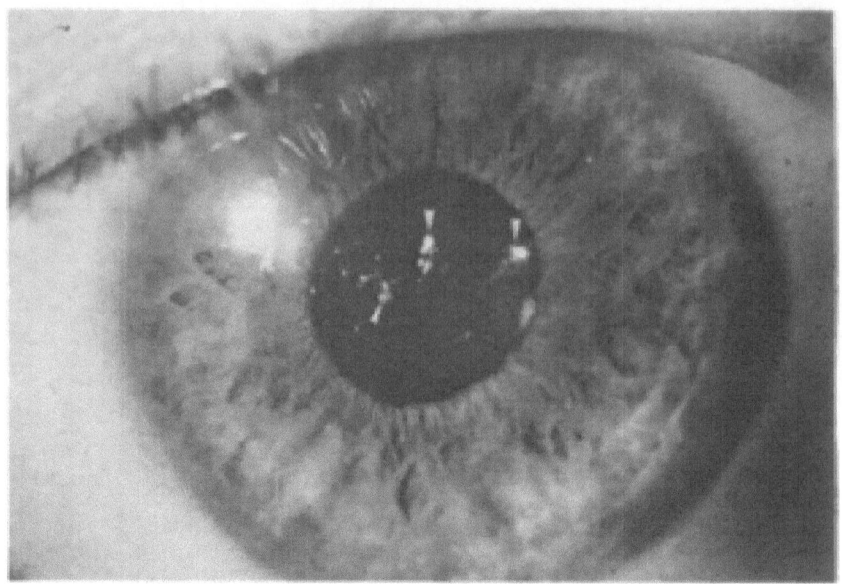

Fig. IX-9. — Mucoid plaques (arrows) in KCS.

Rarely *mucoid plaques* (fig. IX-9) develop on corneal surface in keratoconjunctivitis sicca (Fraunfelder et al., 1977). In one patient, suffering from Sjögren's syndrome, we observed a large honey-comb mucoid plaque on the cornea. Histopathological study by corneal replica technique revealed that the mucoid patch is in fact a mass of degenerated epithelial cells arising in a similar fashion as the corneal filaments (fig. IX-10). Histochemically it contained alcian blue and PAS positive material and degenerated epithelial cells.

Duke-Elder (1965) stated that *indolent ulcers, leucomas and pannus formation* are rare. However, corneal thinning and perforations have been reported especially after topical corticosteroid therapy, which may precipitate corneal thinning and perforation in rheumatoid arthritis and Sjögren's syndrome (Sjögren, 1933 and 1935; Bloch et al., 1965; Gudas et al., 1973; Krachmer and Laibson, 1974).

We have observed dramatic perforation of the cornea in eyes with Sjögren's syndrome. In what way corticosteroids accelerate the corneal thinning and perforation is a matter of conjecture. It is not clear if the dry eye state plays a role in corneal thinning. Brown and Grayson (1968) described marginal furrows in 9 patients suffering from rheumatoid arthritis for at least 5 years with or without keratitis sicca. They also noticed the deleterious effect of corticosteroids in

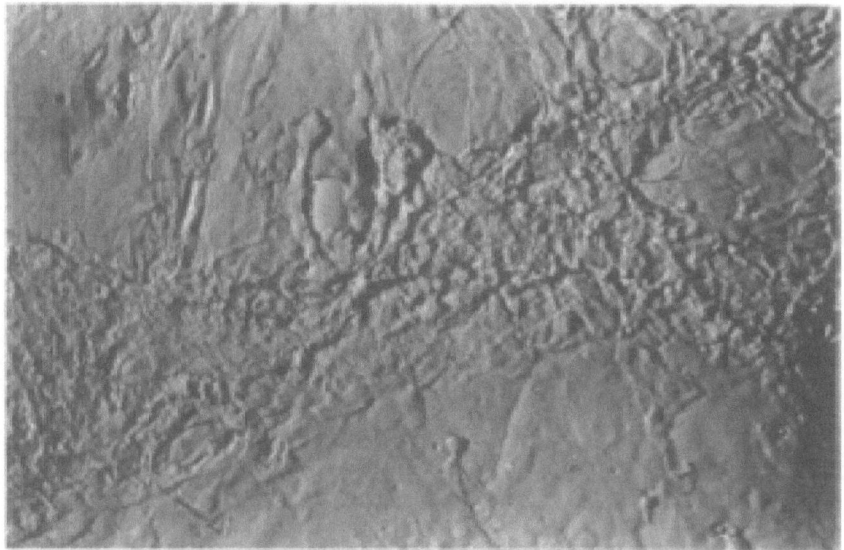

Fig. IX-10. — Histological appearance of the mucoid plaque. Oblique illumination microscopy of the replica. ×180.

some patients. Thus the dryness of the eye may not be directly responsible for patchy corneal thinning. On the other hand patients with keratitis sicca have poor repair capabilities (Dohlman, 1966). In experimental dry eyes (Maudgal and Missotten, 1978), and in patients with keratitis sicca the corneal epithelium healing time is longer than the normal epithelium after a corneal replica.

As the corticosteroids reduce fibroblastic activity, cell infiltration, (Ashton and Cook, 1951) and synthesis of precollagen as well as mucopolysaccharides (Burns, 1963); their use may further inhibit corneal repair, especially in a compromised host (Krachmer and Laibson, 1974). The corneal grafts in such eyes may become repeatedly thinned and melt away (Brown and Grayson, 1968) which indicates that as yet unknown underlying pathophysiological mechanism may play a role in corneal thinning in such patients. Radtke et al. (1978) observed the development of sterile corneal ulcers in patients of keratoconjunctivitis sicca who did not receive any corticosteroid therapy after cataract surgery. The authors emphasize the importance of recognition of dry eye condition prior to surgery, so that the post operative complication may be prevented by vigorous treatment of keratitis sicca.

Microbiology

Staphylococci have been isolated more often from dry eyes of patients (Williamson et al., 1971) and experimental animals (Maudgal, 1976). No viral flora have been detected by immunofluorescence and tissue culture techniques in keratoconjunctivitis sicca (Williamson et al., 1975) or by electron microscopy of experimental dry eyes (Maudgal, 1976).

Diagnostic tests

A. *Evaluation of tear secretory function:* these procedures are designed to estimate roughly the adequacy of aqueous tear secretion.

1. *Marginal tear strip inspection:* in normal eyes the inferior marginal tear strip is continuous, full, slightly concave and about 0,5 mm wide (Dohlman et al., 1970). A deficient or absent tear strip is suggestive of inadequate tear production.

2. *Schirmer test:* first described by Schirmer (1903), this test gives a rough quantitative estimate of tear secretion. In Schirmer I test a Whatman 41 filter paper strip (35 × 5 mm) is folded 5 mm from one end and inserted into the lower fornix over the lower lid margin on its lateral third part. Inserting the folded end over medial third may give slightly higher values due to pooling of tears in this area before their elimination through the punctum.

After 5 minutes the length of the filter paper wetting is measured from the fold. Normal values are 15 mm or more. Values less than 15 mm denote aqueous tear deficiency. Van Bijsterveld (1969), however, suggested 5.5 mm wetting as the division between normal and an abnormally low value. Using this limit only one of six patients would be misclassified. We frequently observe values of Schirmer test between 5 and 10 mm in patients without any keratitis sicca, especially in elderly people.

In *Schirmer II test* the eye is anaesthetized by a topical anaesthetic before performing the test. As the irritation due to filter paper is eliminated this test provides an estimate of basal tear secretion.

Jones (1966) suggested that in performing this test the wetting time should be recorded during 10 minutes or longer to achieve more accurate estimates. In performing this test one should allow the topical anaesthetic to flow out of the cul-de-sac before inserting the filter paper strip. Also the lacrimal drainage system should not be blocked which leads to false high values.

Schirmer III test is the modification of Schirmer II test where the nasal mucosa is irritated by ammonia vapours or cotton wisp during the test to elicite reflex tearing. Reflex tearing may also be stimulated by flashing bright light into the eyes.

The introduction of several variants of Schirmer's test demonstrates that none of them is reliable. There is no correlation between the values of Schirmer test and the severity of keratoconjunctivitis (Scherz et al., 1974; Maudgal, 1976). Also the tear secretion decreases with age in elderly people (de Roeth, 1953).

3. *Dye Dilution tests:* An approximate estimate of tear production can be arrived at by using Norn's dye dilution technique (Norn, 1965a, 1965b, and 1966). Fifty milligrams of fluorescein sodium and rose bengal each and 75 mg of sodium chloride are dissolved in 5 ml distilled water. After instilling one drop of the solution the colour of the lower marginal tear strip is observed with a slitlamp and compared with a dye dilution scale.

Sophisticated dye dilution tests are available for more accurate measurements of tear volume and tear turnover (Maurice. 1963; Mishima et al., 1966) Although these tests demonstrate significantly reduced tear volumes in keratocojunctivitis sicca, they do not correlate well with the severity of rose bengal staining or with the values of Schirmer test (Scherz et al., 1974).

4. *Tear film break up time:* The break up time is measured by staining the tear film with fluorescein and keeping the eye lids apart after blinking. Breaks in the tear film or dry spots appear as dark areas due to lack of fluorescein. The time lapsed between the last blink and the appearance of first dry spot is the break up time. A break up time less than 10 seconds is considered abnormal (Dohlman et al., 1970). Tear film breaks quickly in keratoconjunctivitis sicca due to aqueous or mucus deficiency conditions (Norn, 1969; Brown, 1970, Lemp et al., 1970a and b). In the later condition, however, aqueous tear production may be sufficient (Lemp et al., 1971).

Contrary to the contention of Lemp and Hamill (1973); Vanley et al. (1977) observed that break-up time was not a closely reproducible phenomenon for the normal eye. Therefore, breakup time measurements do not carry any conclusive value but may be helpful as a supportive test in the diagnosis of certain dry eye conditions.

5. *Lysozyme test:* A decrease in the tear lysozyme content in keratoconjunctivitis sicca has been known for over 30 years (Meyer, 1948, Regan, 1950, McEwen and Kimura, 1955). Decreased concentration of lysozyme was found to precede all other symptoms of keratoconjunctivitis sicca (Thygeson and Kimura, 1963). Bonavida and Sapse (1968) and van Bijsterveld (1969) found the measurement of tear lysozyme levels a reliable and most sensitive test for the diagnosis of keratoconjunctivitis sicca. In 1974, van Bijsterveld described a standardized version of the agar diffusion technique for lysozyme determination using commercial medium.

Essentially the test involves the measurement of the zone of lysis of micrococcus lysodeiktious on agar plates in which filter paper discs soaked in tear fluid are placed for 24 hours.

Contrary to the results of Mackie and Seal (1976) who found decreased lysozyme levels in only one out of six patients of keratoconjunctivitis sicca; Avisar et al. (1979) observed significantly lower lysozyme concentration in dry eyes than in control eyes. There was no correlation, however, in the titer of lysozyme in tear fluid and the rate of tear flow.

B. *Evaluation of the corneal epithelium*

1. *Rose Bengal test:* Rose bengal, 1% aqueous solution stains the keratinised cells and mucus whereas fluorescein mixes in the tear fluid accumulated in punctate corneal erosions or the surface irregularities. The corneal staining with rose bengal, however, may not be uniform. It may be localized fine punctate staining of the exposed parts of the cornea and conjunctiva or may diffusely involve the entire corneal surface. Some clinicians and investigators prefer to score the severity of staining by giving a maximum score of 3 each to cornea and the medial and lateral bulbar conjunctiva. However, there is no standardized method of scoring. Rose bengal also stains corneal filaments.

2. *Conjunctival biopsy:* In patients with adequate tear secretion and markedly decreased breakup time conjunctival biopsy from inferior nasal palpebral area may reveal decreased or absent goblet cells in histological sections (Dohlman et al., 1970; Lemp et al., 1971).

3. *Corneal replica:* the corneal replica technique allows the histological examination of superficial epithelium in doubtful or atypical cases (Maudgal and Missotten, 1978; Maudgal et al., 1979). The presence of irregularly arranged, keratinised, partially detached, and piled up cells is typical of keratoconjunctivitis sicca.

Treatment

Treatment of keratoconjunctivitis sicca is essentially symptomatic and directed to combat dryness of the eye, protection of the cornea and elimination of associated infections if present. *Tear substitutes* are artificial preparations administered locally to supplement the natural tear production. Instillation of physiological saline may provide momentary relief but is not of much value as it flows out of the eye in a few minutes (Dohlman et al., 1970). In order to prolong contact time, *viscosity enhancing agents* like methylcellulose and its different polymers (carboxymethylcellulose, hydroxypropylmethylcellulose, hydroxy ethylcellulose) have been employed (Swan, 1945; Mims, 1951; Jones and Coop, 1965; Lemp, 1973). Methylcellulose is sticky, leads to crust formation on the lids and causes increased discomfort in presence of thick mucus in the cul-de-sac. Other polymers of methylcellulose are available in different commercial tear substitutes. Jones and Coop (1965) found that the dry eye patients prefer tear substitutes with higher pH (pH 8.45); a point to be kept in mind in developing different formulations. Also conjunctival mucus dissolves better in alkaline pH giving subjective improvement of symptoms. Polyvinyl alcohol is another polymer unrelated to methylcellulose or its derivatives which also prolongs the contact time of aqueous solutions to the cornea (Krishna and Brow, 1964; Norn, 1977). Artificial tear fluids, in addition, contain inorganic ions for isotonicity and proper pH.

The tear substitutes have to be instilled frequently to give symptomatic relief to the patient. In severe cases one may have to instill artificial tears every 10 minutes or even at shorter intervals. The frequency of instillation is judged by hit and trial method.

We instruct our patients to use the tear drops every one hour to begin with. If the symptoms do not improve the frequency of instillation is increased. On the other hand if the patient feels comfortable, the interval between the drops is increased. The patients should instill the drops regularly. Less benefit is obtained when the tear fluids are instilled only when the patient feels discomfort. Intense therapy stands a better chance to break the vicious circle of irritation-inflammation; and may lead to prolonged periods of well being without treatment.

The antiseptics and preservatives in the commercially available artificial tear fluids produce alterations in the corneal epithelium, as has been stressed recently by Brewitt and Bonatz (1979). Their deleterious effects may outbalance the benefit of the increased fluid in the tear film, especially when the patient has become allergic to one of these substances; a complication likely to occur in chronic treatment.

Keratitis sicca is often associated with blepharitis, and secretions of the palpebral glands, mucoid strands and dried tear substitutes accumulate on the lid margins. Careful and frequent *cleaning of the eyelids and lashes* with dilute boric acid solution is indicated. Alternatively, ordinary household goods like toilet soap or baby shampoo are equally effective for this purpose.

To avoid too frequent instillation of artificial tears, *constant delivery devices* adapted to spectacle frames have been developed (Flynn and Schulmeister, 1967; Dohlman et al., 1971; Ralph et al. 1975). We have experimented with such a modified device. A reservoir is built in the angles and along the arms of the spectacle or goggles frame. From the bottom of the reservoir fluid is lead by means of a thin steel tubing along the lower rim of the frame to the bridge of the nose. Here the steel tubing is fitted with a thin silicone tube which is brought into contact with the medial canthus of the eye. Silicone tube has the advantage that it is not wettable. Therefore the surface tension at the opening of the tube prevents leakage of the fluid. However, if the open end is brought in contact with skin or medial canthus, a slow and constant flow of fluid takes place. This mode of delivery was very effective in a patient, a teacher by profession, with severe keratoconjunctivitis sicca not responding to instillation of artificial tears every 10 minutes or even at shorter intervals.

To reduce aqueous tear evaporation special spectacle or goggle attachments have been designed (Flynn and Schulmeister, 1968). Alternatively, swimmers goggles or protective moist chamber dressings may be used as a temporary measure (MacCarthy and Hollenhorst, 1971; Proirier et al., 1977). These measures, however, interfere in vision due to fogging of the glass. In case of the spectacles and goggles this difficulty may be overcome by covering the glass surface with an antifog coating.

An effective method of natural *tear conservation* is the closure of punctum by electro-cautery. This method should, however, be applied if tear substitutes fail to ameliorate the symptoms in severe cases. Otherwise epiphora may result due to lack of drainage (Jones and Coop, 1965; Jones, 1977; Dohlman, 1978). Temporary occlusion in individual cases by gelatin rod, hydroxyethyl-methacrylate plug or cyanoacrylate adhesives, may be done to assess the benefit of a permanent closure by electro-cautery (Foulds, 1961; Freeman, 1975; Patten, 1976), but these plugs have to be made for individual use as they are not commercially available.

Parotid duct has been transplanted into the conjunctival sac to lubricate the eye with salivary secretions (Charleux and Brun, 1977). However, the procedure has disadvantage of copious flow of fluid into the eye during meals and may aggravate xerostomia in severe cases. The salivary secretions lead to crust formation on the conrea and its enzymatic contents are harmful in keratoplasties.

Acetylcystein 10% or 20% has been employed to *dissolve excess mucus and to treat filamentary keratitis* (Jones and Coop, 1965; Abalson and Brown, 1968; Messner and Leibowitz, 1971; Williamson et al., 1974). Corneal filaments can also be removed by the replica technique (Maudgal et al., 1979). *In mucin deficiency conditions*, on the other hand, one needs to add agents with wetting properties to the artificial tears. Gelatin and synthetic BP-polymer have been found to be usefull in this respect (Holly and Lemp, 1971 a and b; Dohlman, 1971).

The *scleral hard lenses* are helpful in some patients of Stevens-Johnson syndrome and ocular pemphigoid (Ridley, 1963; Gould, 1970). The *acrylate hydrogel soft lenses* are better tolerated (Gasset and Kaufman, 1971). The lenses serve as a type of protective corneal bandage. They have been used in conjunction with copious rinsing, but in spite of great care frequent severe infections have been noted.

Various *systemic drugs* have been tried in an attempt to increase lacrimal secretion. A beneficial effect of topical and systemic bromhexine has been shown in uncontrolled and double blind cross over trials (Neubauer, 1973; Rossmann, 1974; Frost Larsen et al., 1978). Radnot and Follmann (1977) administered a parathyroid extract or synthetic gamma-L-glutamyl-tourin (Litoren) to patients with keratoconjunctivitis sicca. The alleviation of symptoms was accompanied by improvement in the histology and ultrastructure of the corneal and conjunctival epithelium.

Hormonal substitution therapy may be helpful in the post-menopausal female patients. Prijot et al. (1972) recommended the use of estriol (Aacifemine®). We were able to confirm the observations of these authors that in some patients significant improvement of the subjective symptoms may be obtained, without any objective change in tear secretion.

Immunosuppressive therapy may have a role in the treatment of keratoconjunctivitis sicca associated with immunological disorders. Crompton (1968) reported the improvement of Schirmer test values after azathioprine (Immurane®) therapy in a case of lichen planus and another with keratoconjunctivitis sicca who had thyroglobulin antibodies and antibody to gastric parietal cells.

To combat *associated infections,* especially by staphylococci, local antibiotics should be employed. *Corticosteroids* give the feeling of subjective comfort but should be avoided because of the danger of corneal thinning and perforation.

Finally, in the therapeutic considerations of dry eyes, one should not forget the psychological reactions of the patient to this symptomatic condition. In most instances the objective signs of KCS are relatively minor, but the scratchy feeling in the eyes may be incapacitating or only a minor complaint depending on the psychic attitude of the patient.

In patients with marked discomfort, superflous eye examinations by a succession of ophtalmologists; each prescribing a different treatment or just changing the commercial tear substitute preparations, none of which brings relief; may drive a patient to exasperation. The prescription of sedatives may aggravate the situation, although this has not been demonstrated conclusively. It is a common experience, however, that a patient with dry eye complaints is a chronic user of tranquillizers and sedatives.

On the other hand great patience and comprehension, coupled with thoughtful counseling may work wonders. One of our patients with very severe keratitis sicca, in whom we had tried every available treatment, improved markedly with the use of continuous irrigation spectacles. However, when finely we succeeded in constructing a cosmetically acceptable pair, the subjective complaints had improved so much that these spectacles were no longer needed. Although we could not detect any tear secretion by Schirmer test, the complaints of dry eye had almost disappeared and the patient has remained comfortable for years.

Our impression is that attention and compassion had achieved what medication alone could not influence.

In conclusion, medical therapy should include careful cleaning of eyelids and lashes, a search for the tear substitute that provides most comfort to a given patient, and humidification of the air. Short periods of vigorous treatment may bring prolonged subjective improvement.

BIBLIOGRAPHY

Abalson, M.J. and Brown, C.A. — Acetylcysteine in keratoconjunctivitis sicca. *Brit. J. Ophthal.*, *52*, 310, 1968.
Anderson, J.R., Gray, R.G., Beck, J.S. and Kinnear, W.F. — Precipitating autoantibodies in Sjögren's disease. *Lancet*, *2*, 456, 1961.
Appelmans, M. — La keratoconjunctivite sèche de Gougerot-Sjögren. *Arch. Ophtal.*, *8*, 577, 1948.
Ashton, N. and Cook, C. — Effect of cortisone on healing of corneal wounds. *Brit. J. Ophthal.*, *35*, 708, 1951.
Avisar, R., Menache, R., Shaked, P., Rubenstein, J., Machtey, I. and Savir, H. — Lysozyme content of tears in patients with Sjögren's syndrome and rheumatoid arthritis. *Amer. J. Ophthal.*, *87*, 148, 1979.
Baum, J.L., Mishima, S. and Boruchoff, S.A. — On the nature of dellen. *Arch. Ophthal.*, *79*, 657, 1968.
Baum, J.L. — Keratoconjunctivitis sicca. *Trans. Amer. Acad. Ophthal. Otolaryngol.*, *81*, 619, 1976.
Beck, J.S., Anderson, J.R., Bloch, K.J., Buchanan, W.W. and Bunim, J.J. — Antinuclear and precipitating autoantibodies in Sjögren's syndrome. *Ann. Rheum. Dis.*, *24*, 16, 1965.
Bertram, U., Pindborg, J.J., Seedorff, H.H. and Videback, A. — Sjögren's syndrome, with special reference to oral findings. *Ugeskr. Laeg.*, *123*, 1085, 1961.
Bloch, K.J. and Bunim, J.J. — Sjögren's syndrome and its relation to connective tissue diseases. *J. Chr. Dis.*, *16*, 915, 1963.
Bloch, K.J., Buchanan, W.W., Wohl, J.J. et al. — Sjögren's syndrome: A clinical, pathological and serological study of 62 cases. *Medicine*, *44*, 187, 1965.
Bonavida, B. and Sapse, A.T. — Human tear lysozyme II. Quantitative determination with standard schirmer strips. *Amer. J. Ophthal.*, *66*, 70, 1968.
Bowers, D. — Sjögren's syndrome: systemic lupus erythematosus and auto-immune haemolytic anaemia. Report of a case with long survival. *Can. med. Ass. J.*, *100*, 1148, 1969.
Brewitt, H. and Bonatz, E. — Experimentelle Untersuchungen über die Austrocknung des Hornhautepithels. *Read in the symposium on scanning electron microscopy in Ophthalmology*, Brest, June 1979.
Brown, S.I. and Grayson, M. — Marginal furrows. A characteristic corneal lesion of rheumatoid arthritis. *Arch. Ophthal.*, *79*, 563, 1968.
Brown, S.I. — Further studies on the pathophysiology of keratitis sicca of Rollet. *Arch. Ophthal.*, *83*, 542, 1970.
Brown, S.I. — Dry spots and corneal erosions. *Int. Ophthal. Clin.*, *13*, 149, 1973.
Bunim, J.J., Buchanan, W.W., Wertlake, P.T., Sokoloff, L., Bloch, K.J., Beck, J.S. and Alepa, F.P. — Clinical, pathological and serological studies in Sjögren's syndrome. *Ann. Intern. Med.*, *61*, 509, 1964.

Bunim, J.J. — The frequent occurence of hypergammaglobuineuria and multiple tissue antibodies in Sjögren's syndrome. *Ann. N.Y. Acad. Sci., 124,* 852, 1965.

Burns, R.P. — Characteristics of ocular infections agents that are importance in the understanding of eye infections. *In the New Orleans Academy of Ophthalmology symposium on Infectious Diseases of the Conjunctiva and cornea.* St. Louis, C.V. Mosby, 1963.

Charleux, J. and Brun, P. — Traitement chirurgical des syndromès sec oculaires. *Bull. Mem. Soc. Fr. Ophthal., 89,* 177, 1977.

Coverdale, H. — Sjögren's syndrome as a constitutional defect. *N.Z. med. J., 54,* 641, 1955.

Crews, S.J. and Whitfield, A.G.W. — Sjögren's syndrome. *Postgrad. med. J., 39,* 324, 1963.

Crompton, D.O. — Immuno-suppressive drug treatment of keratitis sicca, including an example of lichen planus of the conjunctiva. *Anst. N.Z. J. Surg., 38,* 143, 1968.

De Haas, E.B.H. — Deux complications oculaires rares de la maladie de Bernier-Boeck chez un même sujet. Keratoconjunctivite sèche et calcification de la cornée et de la conjunctive. *Ophthal., 123,* 65, 1952.

Denko, C.W. and Bergenstal — The Sicca Syndrome (Sjögren's syndrome). *Arch. Intern. Med., 105,* 849, 1960.

Denko, C.W. — Antibodies in the Sicca Syndrome (Sjögren's syndrome). *Arthr. and Rheum., 8,* 970, 1965.

de Roeth, A. — Lacrimation in normal eyes. *Arch. Ophthal., 49,* 185, 1953.

Dohlman, C.H. — Corticosteroids in corneal surgery. *Int. Ophthal. Clin., 6,* 845, 1966.

Dohlman, C.H., Lemp, M.A. and English, F.P. — Dry eye syndromes. *Int. Ophthal. Clin., 10,* 215, 1970.

Dohlman, C.H. — New concepts in ocular xerosis. *Trans. Ophthal. Soc. U.K., 91,* 105, 1971.

Dohlman, C.H., Doane, M.G. and Reshmi, C.S. — Mobile infusion pumps for continuous delivery of fluid and therapeutic agents to the eye. *Ann. Ophthal., 3,* 126, 1971.

Dohlman, C.H. — Punctal occlusion in keratoconjunctivitis sicca. *Ophthal., 85,* 1277, 1978.

Duke Elder, S. and MacPaul, P.A. In: System of ophthalmology, Vol. XIII. The ocular adenexa Duke Elder, S. (Ed.) Kimpton, London, 1974, p. 599.

Duke Elder, S. — System of Ophthalmologie. Vol. VIII. Diseases of the other eye. Duke Elder, S. (Ed.) Kimpston, London, 1965, p. 131.

Escande, J.P. and Degos — Les syndromes de Gougerot-Sjögren. *Presse méd., 76,* 1421, 1968.

Feltkamp, T.E.W. and van Rossum, A.L. — Antibodies to salivary duct cells and other idiopathic autoimmune diseases. *Clin. Expt. Immun., 3,* 1, 1968.

Ferreira-Marques, J.A. — Contribution to the study of the Sjögren syndrome. *Acta dermato-venerol (Stockholm)., 40,* 485, 1960.

Flynn, F. and Schulmeister, A. — Keratoconjunctivitis sicca and new techniques in its management. *Med. J. Aust., 1,* 33, 1967.

Flynn, F. and Schulmeister, A. — An improved tear conserving goggle attachment. *Med. J. Aust., 170,* 1968.

Fogel, D.H. — Sjögren's syndrome with benign purpura hyperglobulinaemia. *New Engl. J. Med., 261,* 81, 1959.

Fox, J.T. Jr. — Sjögren's syndrome and late-life myopathy. *Arch. Neurol. (Chicago), 15,* 397, 1966.

Foulds, W.S. — Intracellular gelatin implants in the treatment of keratoconjunctivitis sicca. *Brit. J. Ophthal., 45,* 625, 1961.

François, J., Victoria-Troncoso, V. and Maudgal, P.C. — Keratoconjunctivite sèche expérimentale. (Étude microscopique et histochimique). *Ann. Ocul., 207,* 185, 1974.

François, J., Maudgal, P.C. and Victoria-Troncoso, V. — Experimental keratitis sicca. The corneal epithelium at the transmission and scanning electron microscope. *Ophthal. Res., 8,* 414, 1976.

Fraunfelder, F.T., Wright, P. and Tripathi, R.C. — Corneal mucus plaques. *Amer. J. Ophthal.*, *83*, 191, 1977.
Freeman, J.M. — The punctum plug: Evaluation of a new treatment for the dry eye. *Trans. Amer. Acad. Ophthal. Otolaryngol.*, *79*, 874, 1975.
Frost-Larsen, K., Isager, H. and Manthorpe, R. — Sjögren's syndrome treated with bromhexine: a randomised clinical study. *Brit. Med. J.*, *1*, 1579, 1978.
Gamp, A. — Sjögren's syndrome. *Rheumatism*, *14*, 51, 1958.
Gasset, A.R. and Kaufman, H.E. — Hydrophillic lens therapy of severe keratoconjunctivitis sicca and conjunctival scarring. *Amer. J. Ophthal.*, *71*, 1185, 1971.
Gould, H.L. — The dry eye and scleral contact lenses. *Amer. J. Ophthal.*, *70*, 37, 1970.
Gudas, P.P. Jr., Altman, B., Nicholson, D.H. and Green, R. — Corneal perforation in Sjögren's syndrome. *Arch. Ophthal.*, *90*, 470, 1973.
Guillaine, J., Sterin, D. and Menateau, J.P. — Cryoglobulinaemia with Gougerot-Sjögren's syndrome. *Bull. Soc. Franç. Syph.*, *77*, 751, 1970.
Hardsky, M., Herout, V., Gernik, F., Suzama, L., Rondiakova, Z. and Kvasnicka, J. — Das Gougerot-Houwer-Sjögren syndrom und die polyarteritis nodosa. *Z. Ges. Inn. Med.*, *23*, 25, 1968.
Haye, C., Calle, R. and Cueto-Alvarez — Syndrome de Mikulicz par lymphoreticulosarcome. *Bull. Soc. Belge Ophtal.*, *148*, 390, 1968.
Heaton, J.M. — Sjögren's syndrome and systemic lupus erythematosus. *Brit. Med. J.*, *1*, 466, 1959.
Heindle, I. — Symptomatische Sjögren syndrome nach lymphosarkom. *Derm. Wschr.*, *153*, 536, 1967.
Henderson, J.W. — Keratoconjunctivitis sicca. A review with a survey of 121 additional cases. *Amer. J. Ophthal.*, *33*, 197, 1950.
Holly, F.J. and Lemp, M.A. — Surface chemistry of the tear film; implications for dry eye syndromes, contact lenses and ophthalmic polymers. *Contact lens Soc. Amer. J.*, *5*, 12, 1971 a.
Holly, F.J. and Lemp, M.A. — Wettability and wetting of the corneal epithelium. *Exp. Eye Res.*, *11*, 239, 1971 b.
Holly, F.J. — Formation and rupture of the tear film. *Exp. Eye Res.*, *15*, 515, 1973.
Hood, J., Burns, G.A. and Hodges, R.E. — Sjögren's syndrome in scurvy. *New Engl. J. Med.*, *282*, 1120, 1970.
Horan, E.C. — Ophthalmic manifestations of progressive systemic lupus erythematosus. *Brit. J. Ophthal.*, *53*, 388, 1969.
Hornbaker, J.H. Jr., Foster, E.A., Williams, G.S. and Davis IV J.S. — Sjögren's syndrome and nodular reticulum cell sarcoma. *Arch. Intern. Med.*, *118*, 449, 1966.
Jezegabel, C., Duprey, G. and Rossazza, C. — Syndrome de Mikulicz et leucémie lymphoide. *Rev. oto-neuro-ophtal.*, *38*, 208, 1966.
Jones, L. — The lacrimal secretory system and its treatment. *Amer. J. Ophthal.*, *62*, 47, 1966.
Jones, B.R. and Coop, H.V. — The management of keratoconjunctivitis sicca. *Trans. Ophthal. Soc. U.K..*, *85*, 379, 1965.
Jones, D.B. — Prospects in the management of tear deficiency states. *Trans. Amer. Acad. Ophthal. Otolaryngol.*, *83*, 693, 1977.
Kirkham, T.H. — Scleroderma and Sjögren's syndrome. *Brit. J. Ophthal.*, *53*, 131, 1969.
Kologlu, S. — Un cas de syndrome de Gougerot-Houwer-Sjögren. *Sem. Hôp. Paris*, *34*, 3227, 1958.
Krachmer, J.H. and Laibson, P.R. — Corneal thinning and perforation in Sjögren's syndrome. *Amer. J. Ophthal.*, *78*, 917, 1974.
Krishna, N. and Brow, F. — Polyvinyl alcohol as an ophthalmic vehicle. *Amer. J. Ophthal.*, *57*, 99, 1964.
Kuezynski, A., Evans, R.J.C. and Mitschinson, M.J. — Sicca syndrome due to primary amyloidosis. *Brit. Med. J.*, *2*, 506, 1971.
Kuming, B.S. and Politzer, W.M. — Xerophthalmia and protein malnutritionin in Bantu children. *Brit. J. Ophthal.*, *51*, 649, 1967.

Lehner-Netsch, G., Barry, A. and Delagy, J.M. — Leucémies et maladie auto-immunes: syndrome de Sjögren et anémie hémolytique associés à la leucémies lymphoide chronique. *Canad. Med. Ass. J.*, *24*, 1151, 1969.

Lemp, M.A., Holly, F.J., Iwata, S. and Dohlman, C.H. — The precorneal tear film. Factors in spreading and maintaining a continuous tear film over the corneal surface. *Arch. Ophthal.*, *83*, 89, 1970a.

Lemp, M.A., Dohlman, C.H. and Holly, F.J. — Corneal dessiccation despite normal tear volume. *Ann. Ophthal.*, *2*, 258, 1970b.

Lemp, M.A., Dohlman, C.H., Kuwabara, T., Holly, F.J. and Carroll, J.M. — Dry eye secondary to mucus deficiency. *Trans. Amer. Acad. Ophthal. Otolaryngol.*, *75*, 1223, 1971.

Lemp, M.A. — Tear substitutes in the treatment of dry eyes. *Int. Ophthal. Clin.*, *13*, 145, 1973.

Lemp, M.A. and Hamill, J.R. — Factors affecting tear film breakup in normal eyes. *Arch. Ophthal.*, *89*, 103, 1973.

Leventhal, B.G., Waldorf, D.S. and Talal, N. — Impaired lymphocyte transformation and delayed hypersensitivity in Sjögren's syndrome. *J. Clin. Invest.*, *46*, 1338, 1967.

Marx, E. — De la sensibilité et du desséchement de la cornée. *Ann. Oculist, 158*, 774, 1921.

MacCarthy, C.F. and Hollenhorst, R.W. — Protective moist-chamber eye dressing. *Amer. J. Ophthal.*, *71*, 1333, 1971.

McEwen, W.K. and Kimura, S.J. — Filter paper electrophoresis of tears. *Amer. J. Ophthal.*, *39*, 200, 1955.

Mackie, I.A. and Seal, O.V. — Quantitative tear lysozyme assay in units of activity per microliter. *Brit. J. Ophthal.*, *60*, 70, 1976.

McFarlane, I.G., Wojcicka, B.M., Tsantoulas, D.C., Funk, C., Portmann, B., Eddles-ton, M.L.W.F. and Williams, R. — Cellular immune responses to salivary anti-gens in autoimmune liver disease with sicca syndrome. *Clin. exp. Immunol.*, *25*, 389, 1976.

McLenachan, J. — New aspects of the aetiology of Sjögren's syndrome. *Trans. Ophthal. Soc. U.K.*, *76*, 413, 1956.

Maudgal, P.C. — The epithelial response in keratitis sicca and keratitis herpetica (an experimental and clinical study). Doctoral thesis University of Leuven, 1976. *Doc. Ophthal.*, *45*, 223, 1978.

Maudgal, P.C. and Missotten, L. — Cytology of the superficial keratinised cells in experimental keratitis sicca. *Ophthalmologica*, *176*, 113, 1978.

Maudgal, P.C., Missotten, L. and Van Deuren, H. — Study of filamentary keratitis by replica technique. *Alb. v. Graefes Arch. Klin. exp. Ophthal.*, *211*, 11, 1979.

Maurice, D.M. — New objective fluorophotometer. *Exp. Eye Res.*, *2*, 33, 1963.

Messner, K. and Leibowitz, H.M. — Acetylcysteine treatment of keratitis sicca. *Arch. Ophthal.*, *86*, 357, 1971.

Meyer, K. — Mucopolysaccharides and mucoids of ocular tissues and their enzymatic hydrolysis. In: Sorsby, A. (Ed.), *Modern Trends in Ophthalmology*, Vol. 2, London, Butterworth, 1948.

Mims, J.L. — Methyl cellulose solution for ophthalmic use. *A.M.A. Arch. Ophthal, 46*, 664, 1951.

Mishima, S., Gasset, A., Klyce, S. and Baum, J. — Determination of tear volume and tear flow. *Invest. Ophthal.*, *5*, 264, 1966.

Nagakura, M.M. and Nagakura, M. — A case of Sjögren's syndrome (in Japanese). *J. Otorhinolaryng. Soc. Jap.*, *67*, 1338, 1964.

Neubauer, V.O. — Behandelung der keratoconjunctivitis sicca mit bromhexinhaltigen augentropfen und bromhexine-kapslen. *Wien. Med. Wschr.*, *48*, 719, 1973.

Norn, M.S. — Lacrimal apparatus tests. A new method (lacrimal streak dilution test) Compared with previous methods. *Acta Ophthal. (kbh.)*, *43*, 557, 1965a.

Norn, M.S. — Tear secretion in normal eyes estimated by a new method: the lacrimal streak dilution test. *Acta Ophthal. (kbh.)*, *43*, 567, 1965b.

Norn, M.S. — Tear secretion in diseased eyes. *Acta ophthal. (kbh.)*, *44*, 25, 1966.

Norn, M.S. — Desiccation of the precorneal film: I. Corneal wetting time. *Acta ophthal. (kbh.)*, *47*, 865, 1969.

Norn, M.S. — Treatment of keratoconjunctivitis sicca with liquid paraffin or polyvinyl alcohol in double blind trials. *Acta Ophthal.*, *55*, 945, 1977.

O'Neil, E.M. — Sjögren's syndrome with onset at 10 years of age. *Proc. Royal Soc. Med.*, *58*, 689, 1965.

Paczesniak, R. — A case of Sjögren's syndrome (in Polish). *Klin. Oczna*, *27*, 289, 1957.

Pangrati, D. — Sindrom Sjögren-Gougerot. *Oftal. (Buc.)*, *8*, 231, 1964.

Patten, J.T. — Punctal occlusion with N-butyl cyanoacrylate tissue adhesive. *Ophthal. Surg.*, *7*, 24, 1976.

Pfister, R. and Renner, M. — The histopathology of experimental dry spots and dellen in the rabbit cornea: a light microscopy and scanning and transmission electron microscopy study. *Invest. Ophthal. Vis. Sci.*, *16*, 1025, 1977.

Pittman, F.E. and Holub, D.A. — Sjögren's syndrome and adult coeliac disease. *Gastroenterology*, *48*, 869, 1965.

Proirier, R.H., Ryburn, F.M. and Israel, L.W. — Swimmer's goggles for keratoconjunctivitis sicca. *Arch. Ophthal.*, *95*, 1405, 1977.

Prijot, E., Barzin, L. et Destexhe, B. — Essai de traitement hormonal de la kératoconjonctivite sèche. *Bull. Soc. Belge d'Ophtal.*, *162*, 795-800, 1972.

Radnot, M. and Wallner, E. — Keratoconjunctivitis sicca in Kindersalter. *Ophthal. (Basel)*, *128*, 355, 1954.

Radnot, M. and Follmann, P. — Nouvelle contribution au traitement de la kératoconjunctivite sèche. *Bull. Mém. Soc. Fr. Ophtal.*, *89*, 186, 1977.

Radtke, N., Meyers, S. and Kaufman, H.E. — Sterile corneal ulcers after cataract surgery in keratoconjunctivitis sicca. *Arch. Ophthal.*, *96*, 51, 1978.

Ralph, R.A., Doane, M.G. and Dohlman, C.H. — Clinical experience with a mobile ocular perfusion pump. *Arch. Ophthal.*, *93*, 1039, 1975.

Ramage, J.H., Kinnear, W.F. — Keratoconjunctivitis sicca and the collagen diseases. *Brit. J. Ophthal.*, *40*, 416, 1956.

Regan, E.F. — The lysozyme content of tears. *Amer. J. Ophthal.*, *33*, 600, 1950.

Remolar, J.M., Roisenblit, A. and Brown, L.N. — Syndrome de Sjögren asociado a tiroiditis cronica. *Rev. Asoc. méd. Argent*, *79*, 106, 1965.

Ridley, F. — Scleral contact lenses. *Arch. Ophthal.*, *70*, 740, 1963.

Rossmann, H. — B: Behandlung verminderter tranensekretion mit bromhexin-augentroppen. *Dtsch. Med. Wschr.*, *99*, 408, 1974.

Rozenblit, J. and Tenezynska, I. — A borderline case of Felty's syndrome and Sjögren's syndrome (in Polish). *Wiad. Lek.*, *18*, 1261, 1965.

Scherz, W., Doane, M.G. and Dohlmann, C.H. — Tear volume in normal eyes and keratoconjunctivitis sicca. *Alb. v. Graefes Arch. Klin. Ophthal.*, *192*, 141, 1974.

Schirmer, O. — Studien zur physiologie und pathologie de tränenabsonderung und tränenabfuhr. *Alb. v. Graefes Arch. Klin. Exp. Ophthal.*, *56*, 197, 1903.

Shearn, M.A. and Tu, W.H. — Nephrogenic diabetes insipidus and other defects of renal tubular function in Sjögren's syndrome. *Amer. J. Med.*, *39*, 312, 1965.

Shioji, R., Furyama, T., Onodera, S., Saito, H., Ito, H. and Sasaki, Y. — Sjögren's syndrome and renal tubular acidosis. *Amer. J. Med.*, *48*, 456, 1970.

Sjögren, H. — Zur kenntnis der keratoconjunctivitis sicca: keratitis filiformis bei hypofunktion der tranendrüsen. *Acta Ophthal. Suppl.*, *2*, 1, 1933.

Sjögren, H. — Zur kenntnis der keratoconjunctivitis sicca: II. Algemeine symptamatologie und ätiologie. *Acta Ophthal.*, *13*, 1, 1935.

Sood, N.N. — Sjögren's syndrome (a clinico-pathological study). *J. All India Ophthal. Soc.*, *16*, 19, 1968.

Stanworth, A. — Keratoconjunctivitis sicca. *Brit. J. Ophthal.*, *35*, 317, 1951.

Steinberg, A.D. and Talal, N. — The co-existence of Sjögren's syndrome and systemic lupus erythematosus. *Ann. Intern. Med.*, *74*, 55, 1971.

Stoltze, C.A., Hanlon, D.G., Pease, G.L., Henderson, J.W. — Keratoconjunctivitis sicca and Sjögren's syndrome. Systemic manifestations and haematologie and protein abnormalities. *Arch. Intern. Med. (Chicago)*, *106*, 513, 1960.

Swan, K.C. — The use of methyl cellulose in ophthalmology. *Arch. Ophthal.*, *33*, 378, 1945.

Talal, N. and Bunim, J.J. — The development of malignant lymphoma in the course of Sjögren's syndrome. *Amer. J. Med.*, *36*, 529, 1964.

Thygeson, P. and Kimura, S.J. — Chronic conjunctivitis. *Trans. Amer. Acad. Ophthal. Otolaryngol.*, *67*, 494, 1963.
van Bijsterveld, O.P. — Diagnostic tests in the sicca syndrome. *Arch. Ophthal.*, *82*, 10, 1969.
van Bijsterveld, O.P. — The lysozyme agar diffusion test in he sicca syndrome. *Ophthal.*, *167*, 429, 1973.
van Bijsterveld, O.P. — Standardization of the lysozyme test for a commercially available medium. *Arch. Ophthal.*, *91*, 432, 1974.
Vanley, T., Leopold, I.R. and Gregg, T.H. — Interpretation of tear film break up. *Arch. Ophthal.*, *95*, 445, 1977.
Vanselow, N.A., Dodson, V.N., Angell, D.C. and Duff, J.F. — A clinical study of Sjögren's syndrome. *Ann. Intern. Med.*, *58*, 124, 1963.
Walser, A., Ivankovic, I. and Baur, M. — Sjögren-syndrome und struma lymphomatosa Hashimoto. *Schweiz. med. Wschr.*, *95*, 763, 1965.
Wegelius, O., Fyhrquist, F., Ander, P.L. — Sjögren's syndrome associated with vitamin B_{12} deficiency. *Acta rheum. Scand.*, *16*, 184, 1970.
Williamson, J., Paterson, R.W.W., McGavin, D.D.M., Greig, W.R., Whaley, K. — Sjögren's syndrome in relation to pernicious anaemia and idiopathic Addisonian disease. *Brit. J. Ophthal.*, *54*, 31, 1970.
Williamson, J., Wilson, J., Wallace, J. and Whaley, K. — Studies of the bacterial flora in keratoconjunctivitis sicca. *Eye Ear, Nose, Throat Monthly, 50,* 257, 1971.
Williamson, J., Doig, W.M., Forrester, J.V., Tham, M.H., Wilson, T., Whaley, K. and Dick, W.C. — Management of the dry eye in Sjögren's syndrome. *Brit. J. Ophthal.*, *58*, 798, 1974.
Williamson, J., Doig, W.M., Forrester, J.V., Dick, W.C. and Whaley, K. — Studies of the viral flora in keratoconjunctivitis sicca. *Brit. J. Ophthal.*, *59*, 45, 1975.

CHAPTER X

MARGINAL KERATITIS

Marginal corneal ulcers are frequently associated with conjunctivitis. Corneal periphery may be involved by direct encroachment of conjunctival disease. In other cases marginal keratitis may be a manifestation of metabolic and metastic or allergic manifestation of systemic disease (Duke-Elder and Leigh, 1965).

In this chapter we shall consider staphylococcal blepharoconjunctivitis which produces keratitis on the lower third of the cornea, and the superior limbic keratoconjunctivitis of Theodore, which affects the upper part of the cornea. Marginal catarrhal, metastatic or allergic ulcers and the superficial marginal keratitis of Fuchs, an uncommon condition, which may develop into ring ulcers (Duke-Elder and Leigh, 1965) are not dealt with here.

STAPHYLOCOCCAL BLEPHAROCONJUNCTIVITIS

Staphylococcal infection is the most common cause of blepharitis (Duke-Elder and Leigh, 1965; Locatcher-Khorazo and Seegal, 1972; Smolin and Okumoto, 1977; Fedukowicz, 1978; Newell, 1978; Grayson, 1979).

Staphylococcus aureus causes an ulcerative blepharitis with hard crust formation around the cilia. Staphylococi may be secondary invaders in scaly blepharitis which is primarily seborrheic. Both types may become chronic persisting or recurring for years.

Chronic staphylococcal blepharitis is always accompanied by conjunctivitis. Epithelial keratitis of fine punctate type, especially on the lower third of the cornea, may develop. Punctate erosions, catarrhal ulcers, phlyctenular lesions or stromal infiltrates are not uncommon.

Scrapings of the conjunctiva usually do not show any microorganisms. Keratoconjunctivitis is thaught to be the result of allergic reaction to the bacterial exotoxin (Duke-Elder and Leigh, 1965; Locatcher-Khorazo and Seegal, 1972).

Treatment

The eyelids should be cleaned with hot water compresses. A baby shampoo may be employed for this purpose. Meibomian gland secretions should be mechanically expressed out. After cleaning an antibiotic ointment should be applied to the lid margins and into the eye. Grayson (1979) advised the use of bacitracin, erythromycin and chloramphenicol in the order of preference.

Zinc oxide-ichtyol, yellow oxide of mercury oinments may be used for the same purpose.

SUPERIOR LIMBIC KERATOCONJUNCTIVITIS

Superior limbic keratoconjunctivitis (SLKC), first described by Theodore (1963) is a specific clinical disorder of unknown etiology, characterized by the recurring inflammation of the superior bulbar and tarsal conjunctiva. According to Theodore (1967 and 1971) incidence of SLKC is somewhat greater in females. In the series of Wright (1972) about half of the patients were women while the patients of Corwin (1968); Cher (1969), and Donshik et al. (1978) were predominantly women. The disease is usually bilateral but the clinical condition may be more pronounced in one eye. The disease has been reported in patients from 4 to 81 years age (Theodore and Ferry, 1970); but on reviewing the literature we found the peak incidence in the fourth and fifth decades of life. Corwin (1968) pointed out that till then all the cases reported were sporadic; a fact which remains true to date. The two female patients in Corwin's series were mother and daughter but their initial symptoms appeared at different time intervals.

Apart from this solitary example, there are no reports in literature suggestive of the familial or contagious nature of this disease.

Tenzel (1968) first pointed out the occurrence of elevated protein-bound iodine levels in patients with SLKC. Soon after, Cher (1969) reported that five of his ten patients had thyrotoxicosis or had undergone treatment for hyperthyroidism. Sutherland (1969) reported another patient with thyrotoxicosis. Twenty six percent of Wrights patients (1972) had thyroid disease while Fells (1972) noted that 40%

of patients having dysthyroid exophthalmos developed SLKC. Some patients may have hypothyroidism (Theodore 1968). Symptoms of SLKC may precede the symptoms of hyperthyroidism as two patients of Wright (1972) saught treatment for SLKC in whom thyrotoxicosis was discovered on examination.

Dralands has pointed out that many of her young patients with SLKC have a fine textured pale skin and blond hair (Dralands, L. 1978, personnal communication). To our knowledge, this association with SLKC has not yet been described.

Clinical picture

Characteristically, the patient complains of intense burning or hot feeling under the upper eyelid with pain, foreign body sensation and photophobia. Some patients may complain of an extremely painfull foreign body under the upper eyelid (Corwin, 1968). There is some watery or mucoid discharge. The symptoms vary in severity from week to week; characterized by remissions and exacerbations for prolonged periods (Wright, 1972).

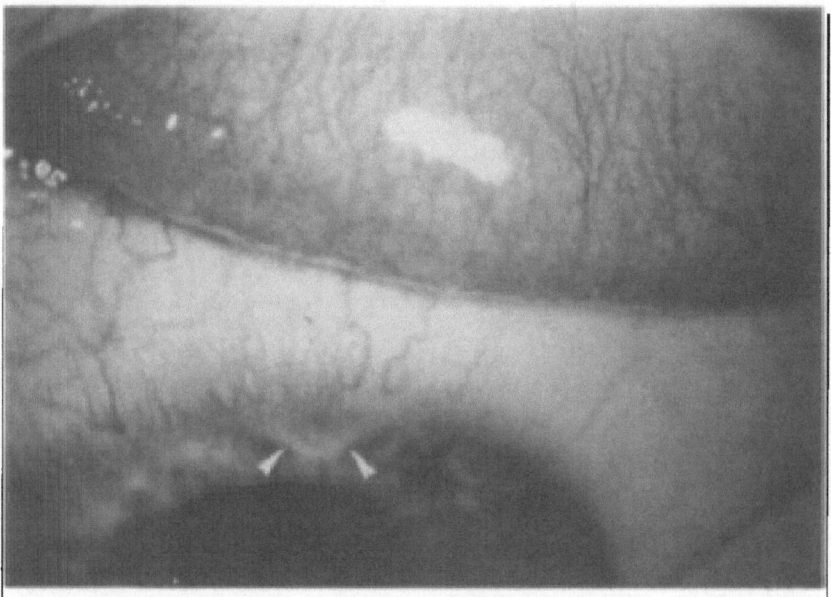

Fig. X-1. — Superior limbic keratoconjunctivitis showing papillary changes on the upper tarsal conjunctiva, limbal congestion and edema, and the corneal involvement (arrows).

On examination, there is slight swelling of the upper eyelid with blepharospasm simulating ptosis in severe cases. In one of Cher's patients (1969), congestive blepharoptosis replaced thyrotoxic lid retraction after the control of toxic state. Papillary conjunctivitis exclusively involves the tarsal conjunctiva of the upper eyelid (figs. X-1), but the degree of tarsal inflammation varies according to the severity of limbal reaction or vice versa. The limbal changes remain limited to the area covered by the upper lid; therefore extending symmetrically from 10 to 2 o'clock positions along the superior corneo-scleral limbus. The inflammed area shows conjunctival as well as deep ciliary congestion (figs. X-1 and X-2). The involved conjunctiva appears corrugated and heaped up, sometimes forming a veritable roll of thickened, fleshy, hypertrophic tissue which might even encroach upon the cornea (Cher, 1969).

The edematous changes and vascular congestion diminish posteriorly but may extend upto the insertion of superior rectus muscle in an arcuate fashion. The edematous change is quite different from chemosis. The involved conjunctiva loses its normal glistening appearance.

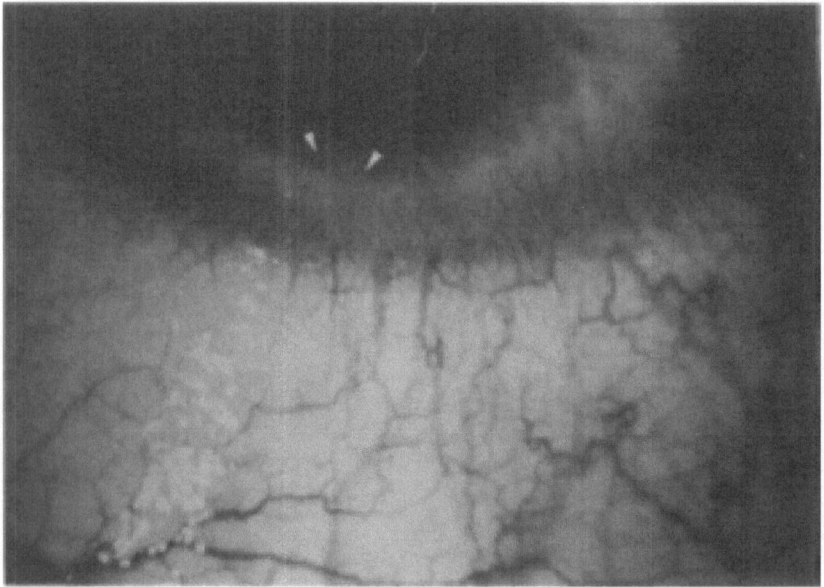

Fig. X-2. — Superior limbic keratoconjunctivitis. The bulbar conjunctiva is corrugated, edematous (scatterred light reflex) and injected. Arrows point to the punctate lesions on the cornea.

In severe cases superficial corneal edema may be present adjacent to the swollen limbal conjunctiva (figs. X-1 and X-2). In mild cases, however, patches of fine punctate keratitis near the superior limbus may become visible only after fluorescein or rose bengal staining. Similar staining occurs on the involved conjunctiva but is most apparent on the swollen limbal area.

Corneal filaments develop in about one third (Theodore, 1967) to half of the cases (Corwin, 1968) and are typically situated in the upper third of the cornea.

There is some sticky mucus in the cul-de-sac but the results of Schirmer test are normal. The lower conjunctival fornix remains unaffected.

The condition runs an unpredictable course. Resolution may occcur suddenly after prolonged unsuccessful treatment or even spontaneously. Recurrences may be just as sudden (Cher, 1969).

Pathology

Scrapings of the involved conjunctiva show keratinised epithelial cells with degenerated nuclei (Theodore and Ferry, 1970).

Light microscopy of the conjunctival tissue shows superficial cornification of the thickened epithelium. Some cells are vacuolated while others are separated by intercellular edema. The subconjunctival tissue is edematous with minimal cellular infiltration (Cher, 1969). These findings have been confirmed and further extended by the histological and ultrastructural studies recently (Collin et al., 1978 a and b; Donshik et al., 1978). The main disturbance is the keratinization of the conjunctival epithelium with development of intracellular keratohyaline granules, accumulation of intracellular glycogen particles and degeneration of nuclei. Donshik et al. (1978) did not find increased inflammatory cell infiltration as compared to control specimens but the lymph vessels were grossly dilated. These authors also did not find keratinization of tarsal conjunctiva in one specimen examined. The goblet cell population was not altered. On the contrary, Wright (1972) found markedly increased number of goblet cells in palpebral conjunctiva. No indication of a viral, bacterial or fungal infection has been seen in any histological or ultrastructural study.

Treatment

Theodore (1967) originally advocated treatment of SLKC by painting the tarsal conjunctiva with 0,5% silver nitrate solution. Finding this treatment ineffective, Cher (1969) and Wright (1972) suggested the use of topical acetylcysteine or 1% adrenaline; mechanical scraping of the tarsal conjunctiva, and soft contact lenses.

These measures, however, have given variable results. Corwin (1968) reported dramatic improvement of punctate keratitis after topical corticosteroid therapy, but the response of limbal changes was not uniform. In the experience of Dralands (1978; personnal communication), subconjunctival injections of depot corticosteroids have consistently lead to the amelioration of the signs and symptoms of SLKC. Recurrences, however, take place. Donshik et al (1978) reported good results after resection of the superior limbal conjunctiva. Resection of the tarsal conjunctiva lead to only temporary improvement.

BIBLIOGRAPHY

Cher, I. — Clinical features of superior limbic keratoconjunctivitis in Australia. *Arch. Ophthal., 82,* 580, 1969.
Collin, H. B., Donshik, P. C., Boruchoff, S. A., Foster, C. S. and Cavanagh, H. D. — The fine structure of nuclear changes in superior limbic keratoconjunctivitis. *Invest. Ophthal. Vis. Sci., 17,* 79, 1978 a.
Collin, H. B., Donshik, P. C., Foster, C. S., Boruchoff, S. A. and Cavanagh, H. D. — Keratinization of the bulbar conjunctival epithelium in superior limbic keratoconjunctivitis in humans. An electron microscopic study. *Acta Ophthal., 56,* 531, 1978 b.
Corwin, M. E. — Superior limbic keratoconjunctivitis. *Amer. J. Ophthal., 66,* 338, 1968.
Donshik, P. C., Collin, H. B., Foster, C. S., Cavanagh, H. D. and Boruchoff, S. A. — Conjunctival resection treatment and ultrastructural histopathology of superior limbic keratoconjunctivitis. *Amer. J. Ophthal., 85,* 101, 1978.
Duke-Elder, S. and Leigh, A. G. — System of ophthalmology. Vol. VIII. Diseases of the outer eye. Part 2. Henry Kimpton, London, 1965.
Fedukowicz, H. B. — External infections of the eye. Appelton-Century-Crafts, N.Y. 1978.
Fells, P. — Discussion on superior limbic keratoconjunctivitis. *Trans. Ophthal. Soc. U.K., 92,* 560, 1972.
Grayson, M. — Diseases of the cornea. The C.V. Mosby Company, St. Louis, 1979.
Locatcher-Khorazo, D. and Seegal, B. C. — Microbiology of the eye. C.V. Mosby Company, St. Louis, 1972.
Newell, F. W. — Ophthalmology, Principles and concepts. The C.V. Mosby Company, St. Louis, 1978.
Smolin, G. and Okumoto, M. — Staphycoloccal blepharitis. *Arch. Ophthal., 95,* 812, 1977.
Sutherland, A. L. — Superior limbic keratoconjunctivitis. Report of a case. *Trans. Ophthal. Soc. N.Z., 21,* 89, 1969.
Tenzel, R. R. — Comments on superior limbic filamentous keratitis. Part 2. *Arch. Ophthal., 79,* 508, 1968.

Theodore, F. H. — Superior limbic keratoconjunctivitis. *Eye Ear Nose Throat Month,* *42,* 25, 1963.

Theodore, F. H. — Further observations on superior limbic keratoconjunctivitis. *Trans. Amer. Acad. Ophthal. Otolaryngol., 71,* 341, 1967.

Theodore, F. H. — Comments on findings of elevated protein bound iodine in superior limbic keratoconjunctivitis. Part 1. *Arch. Ophthal., 79,* 508, 1968.

Theodore, F. H. — Superior limbic keratoconjunctivitis. Further studies. In: *XXI concilium Ophthalmologicum Acta Mexico 1970,* Excerpta Medica, Amsterdam, 1971.

Theodore, F. H. and Ferry, A. P. — Superior limbic keratoconjunctivitis. Clinical and pathological correlations. *Arch. Ophthal., 84,* 481, 1970.

Wright, P. — Superior limbic keratoconjunctivitis. *Trans. Ophthal. Soc. U.K., 92,* 555, 1972.

CHAPTER XI

MANAGEMENT OF SUPERFICIAL KERATITIS

Two factors are of paramount importance in the management of superficial keratitis. Firstly the ophthalmologist should be aquainted with clinical aspect of the disease. A presumptive diagnosis is often sufficient to institute therapy. This may work well in keratitis due to bacterial infections as broad-spectrum and potent specific antibiotics are available. The typical and resistant cases, and disorders due to virus or fungi, however, pose problems where one needs to resort to laboratory tests. The second important factor, therefore, is the ability to prepare smears and to interpret the microscopic findings. If the ophthalmologist is unable to examine the smears, help of a cytologist should be saught. This will usually give the clue to the etiology.

Table XI-1 gives a few guidelines for the study of corneal and conjunctival smears.

TABLE IX-1. — *Interpretation of smears in keratoconjunctivitis*

Cytology	Keratinised cells:	Superior limbic keratoconjunctivitis. Keratoconjunctivitis sicca.
	Inclusion bodies:	Viral and Chlamydial infections.
	Inflammatory cell response:	
	Polymorphoneutrophils	Bacterial, fungal and Chlamydia infections.
	Mononuclear leukocytes	Viral infections.
	Eosinophils	Allergic disorders.
Micro-organisms	Bacteria	Gram + or Gram −
	Fungi	Filamentous or globular.

In addition corneal replicas should be made when keratitis is present. The latter method provides a detailed histological picture of the lesion in superficial keratitis.

CAUSATIVE THERAPY

Bacterial infections

If bacterial infection is present (presumptive diagnosis on the basis of clinical examination and smears) cultures should be done to identify the offending bacteria and to test their sensitivity to antibiotics. In the meantime a broad spectrum topical antibiotic like chloramphenicol, neomycin or one of the tetracyclines should be applied into the eye. This blanket therapy would control many of the Gram positive and Gram negative bacteria. On the basis of sensitivity tests, specific therapy, if available, should be instituted in place of the blanket therapy. The reader should refer to the standard text and reference books for the treatment of specific bacterial keratoconjunctivitis and for detailed description of antibiotic treatment.

Viral infections

Antiviral chemotherapy is available only for herpes simplex and to some extent vaccinia keratitis. However, epithelial dendritic ulcers respond equally well to mechanical abrasions and chemotherapy. In our hands corneal replicas have given excellent therapeutic results in patients resistant to IDU or showing drug reactions. Ara-A is as effective as IDU. Its use is mainly indicated in IDU resistant strains. TFT is more effective than IDU and penetrates the corneal stroma on topical application. Two newly developed promising compounds—acycloguanosine and BVDU—are still at experimental stage. In our experience BVDU is significantly better than IDU in treating experimental herpes simplex epithelial keratitis (Maudgal et al., 1979 and 1980), effective in patients resistant to IDU or Ara-A therapy and significantly better than TFT in the treatment of experimental stromal keratitis, if therapy is begun immediately after inoculation of the virus (unpublished).

The choice of therapy in herpetic dendritic ulcers is also dictated by the location of the lesions. A central ulcer should be treated by the most effective rapid method to avoid stromal infiltrate development. Mechanical abrasion or replica of the epithelium is preferred since it is difficult to predict the effect of antiviral therapy.

The various modes of therapy employed in different forms of viral keratitis are summarized in table XI-2.

TABLE XI-2. — *Treatment of viral keratoconjunctivitis*

Condition	Site/type of lesion	Treatment
Herpes simplex	Conjunctiva	Antiviral agents (IDU, Ara-A, TFT, BVDU*, acycloguanosine).
	Corneal dendritic/or punctate lesions	
	a. central	corneal replica, abrasion (antiviral agents usually not required)
	b. peripheral	Antiviral agents. If deteriorates or does not respond within 48 hours make corneal replica or abrade.
	Corneal dendritic or punctate lesions + stromal involvement	Corneal replica/abrasion to heal epithelial disease. TFT and BVDU* may be used for stromal keratitis. Add corticosteroids only if stromal disease deteriorates.
	Stromal keratitis	Antiviral agents (TFT and BVDU* are prefered) and topical corticosteroids.
Herpes zoster	Conjunctivitis	No treatment required
	Epithelial punctate keratitis	Spontaneous resmission occurs in about 1 week. BVDU* may be used.
	Dendritic lesions	Corneal replica/abrasion. BVDU* may be used.
	Stromal keratitis	Local corticosteroids usually for long periods. BVDU* may be used.
Adenovirus	Keratoconjunctivitis	No specific treatment (Virustat? Corticosteroids?) Corneal replicas prevent the development of stromal opacities.
Warts	Usually lid margin	Removal of the lesion
Molluscum contagiosum	Usually lid margin	Removal of the lesion

* After this report was written we have found that BVDU is effective in all forms of herpes simplex or herpes zoster keratitis, and has been administered orally to a small number of varicella-zoster patients without serious side-effects.

Chlamydia infections

Chlamydia are sensitive to tetracyclines, sulfonamides and Rifampin. Local therapy alone may be effective in trachoma while it gives variable results in TRIC agents keratoconjunctivitis which require systemic therapy (Dawson, 1973).

Fungal infections

Nystatin and flucytosin topical drops are effective against yeastlike fungi. Both of these drugs were effective in curing our patients with Thygeson's superficial punctate keratitis. One percent solution of these drugs, however, has to be instilled every hour for long periods (3 to 6 weeks).

Amphotercine B, Natamycin (Pimafucin®) are effective against filamentous fungi. Pimafucin is however, more effective and better tolerated. New antifungal imidazole compounds (clotrimazole, miconazole, econazole) are not available in Belgium.

Diseases of non-infective or unknown etiology: the preferred modes of treatment of the superficial keratitis in our clinic are given in table XI-3.

TABLE XI-3. — *Treatment of the diseases of non-infective or unknown etiology*

Ocular condition	Treatment
Recurrent corneal erosions	Corneal replica
Persistent epithelial defect (asceptic)	Rinsing therapy
Filamentary keratitis	Corneal replica, mechanical removal, Alum 1%, Acetylcystein 10-30%
Keratonconjunctivitis sicca	Tear substitutes (continuous delivery systems in severe cases)
Superior limbic keratoconjunctivitis	Subconjunctival injection of depot corticosteroids (Celestone Chronadose®)

Role of corticosteroids

Corticosteroids are used in ophthalmology because of their antiinflammatory property. However, topical therapy inhibits fibroblastic and collagen forming activity, may retard epithelial and endothelial regeneration, increases collagenase activity in corneal wounds, promotes the growth of bacteria (Havener, 1978) and fungi, causes penetration of viruses into the cornea, reduces the outflow of aqueous humor and causes development of cataracts.

Because of these deleterious effects corticosteroids should be used with caution. Their ability to prevent inflammatory response and scar formation may help in preventing or reducing corneal opacification and thus restorating useful vision.

However, great skill coupled with personal experience and a close watch over the patient are needed to guide the ophthalmologist in his decisions: when to start local steroids and when to withdraw them; when to increase or to decrease the dosages, and how to wean the corticodependent cornea. Some guidelines have been given in each chapter, but much is left to the art of healing.

Effects of topical ophthalmic drugs on corneal epithelium

Most ophthalmic preparations produce alterations of the corneal epithelium. IDU is toxic in tissue culture systems, and it may have a similar effect on normal corneal epithelium.

Chloramphenicol causes loss of microvilli and roughening of corneal surface (Mitsui et al. 1976). Topical prednisolone instillation not only causes loss of microvilli but also cell membrane destruction (Takashima, 1975). Moreover, the commercially available ophthalmic drugs contain vehicle base and preservatives some of which, like benzalkonium chloride may be potentially toxic to the corneal epithelium (Pfister and Burstein, 1976). We examined the effects of commercially available ophthalmic corticosteroid (Maxidex®), antibiotic (Statrol®) preparations alone or in combination (Chibro-Cadron®, Maxitrol® and De Icol®) on rabbit corneal epithelium by scanning electron microscopy. Instillation of 1 drop of each collyrium 5 times a day for 4 days produced epithelial damage. Loss of microvilli, cell membrane destruction occurred in all eyes (fig. XI-1). Focal areas of exfoliation were also present.

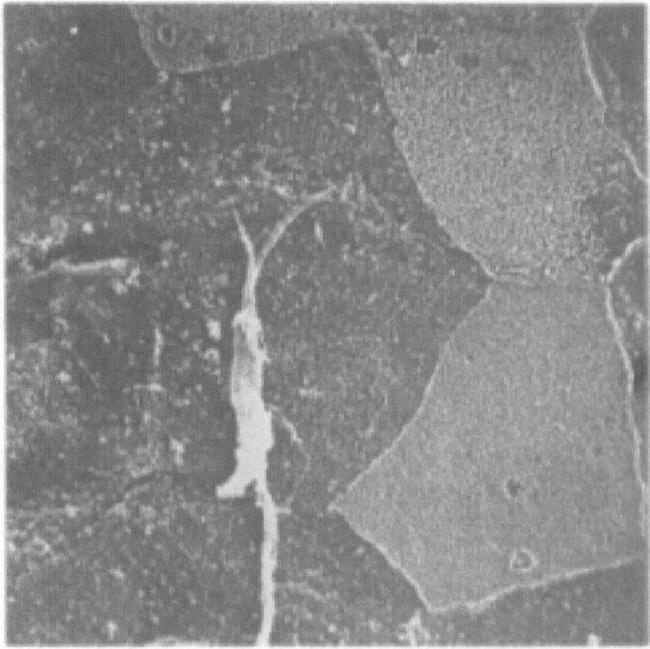

Fig. XI-1. — Loss of microvilli (dark cells), and exfoliation of superficial epithelium after DeIcol® administration in rabbit eye. Scanning electron microscopy. × 1000.

The addition of local anesthetics to some preparations aggravates their toxicity. Prolonged use of any drug may lead to hypersensitivity.

These observations indicate that prolonged and over enthusiastic treatment could produce more damage to the epithelium than the benefit derived from it. As a conclusion one should prescribe drugs only when there is clear-cut indication for their use.

FURTHER READING

Havener, W. H. — Ocular pharmacology, The C.V. Mosby Company, St. Louis, 1978.
Aronson, S. B. and Elliott, J. H. — Ocular inflammation. The C.V. Mosby Company, St. Louis, 1972.

BIBLIOGRAPHY

Dawson, C. — Therapy of diseases caused by chlamydia organisms. External ocular diseases: Diagnosis and current therapy. *Int. Ophthal. Clin.*, *13*, 93, 1973.
Maudgal, P.C., De Clercq, E., Descamps, J., Missotten, L. et al. — (E)-5-(2-bromovinyl)2'-deoxyuridine in the treatment of experimental herpes simplex keratitis. *Antimicrob. Agents Chemother*, *17*, 8, 1980.
Maudgal, P.C., De Clercq, E., Descamps, J. and Missotten, L. — Evaluation of BVDU for the treatment of experimental herpes simplex keratitis. *Bull. Soc. Belge d'Ophtal.*, *186*, 109, 1979b.
Mitsui, Y., Takashima, R., Fujimoto, M. and Kishiyama, T. — Deposits of mucosubstances on the cornea by topical chloramphenicol: an electron microscopic study. *Invest. Ophthal.*, *15*, 211, 1976.
Pfister, R.R. and Burstein, N. — The effects of ophthalmic drugs, vehicles, and preservatives on corneal epithelium: a scanning electron microscope study. *Invest. Ophthal.*, *15*, 246, 1976.
Takashima, R. — Corticosteroid effects on the corneal surface of rabbits studied by scanning electron microscopy. *Jap. J. Ophthal.*, *19*, 393, 1975.

T 2994 Imprimé en Belgique par Ceuterick s.a.
Brusselse straat 153 B 3000-Louvain
A. Struyf Oude Baan 353 B 3040-Korbeek-Lo